closet smarts

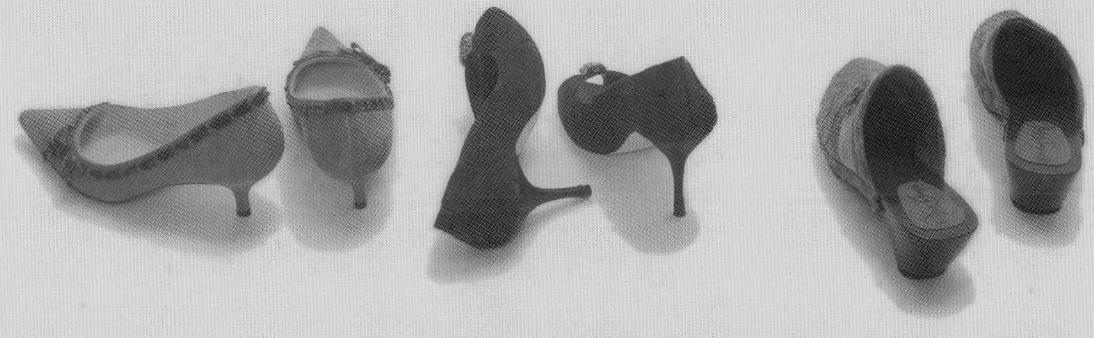

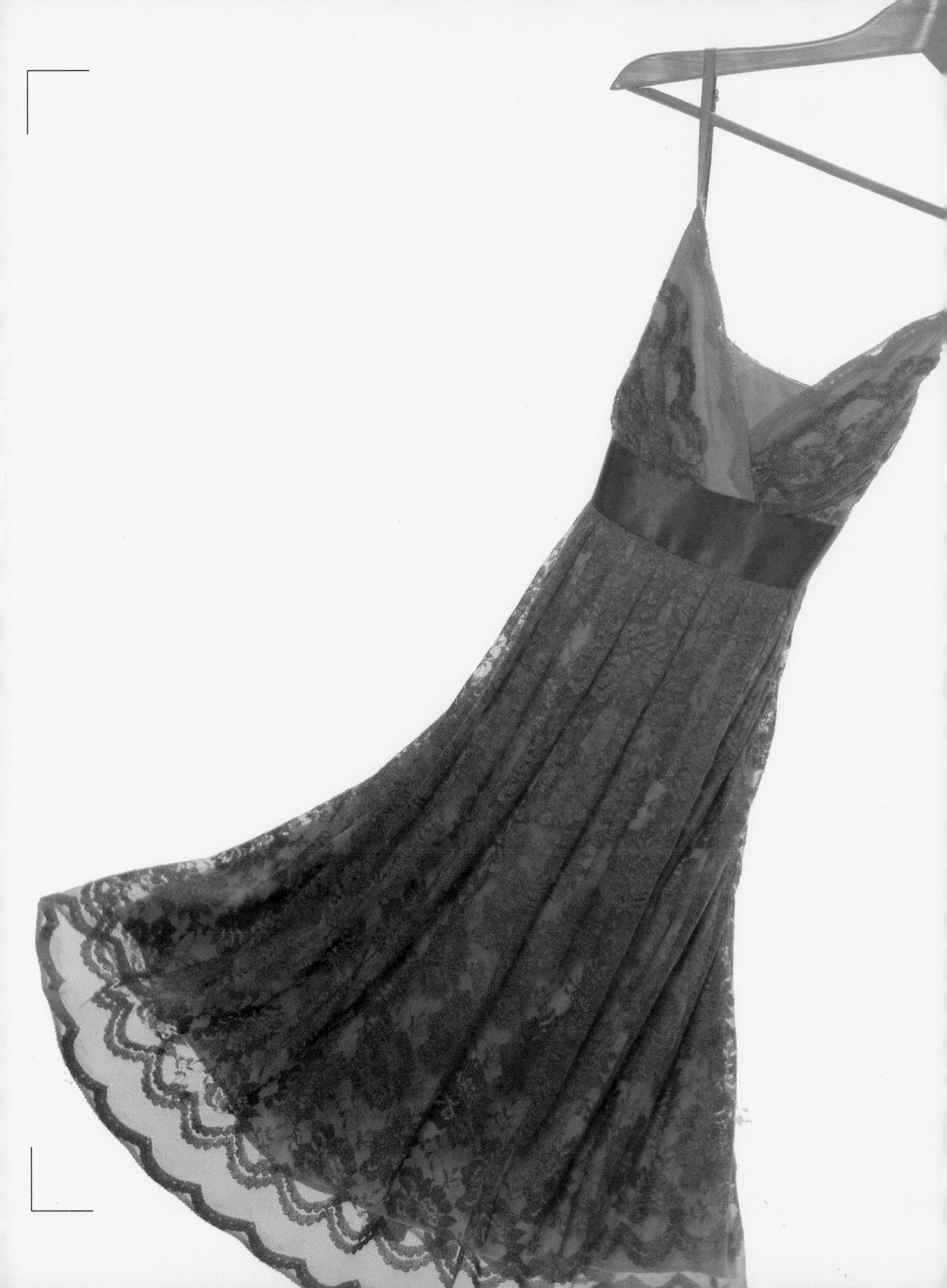

closet smarts

- Find flattering fashions that don't cost a fortune
- Revamp your closet: what to keep, what to toss, what to wear with what
- Clothes you should *never* wear—and why
- Fill wardrobe gaps
- The truth about color, clothes, and you

EMILY NEILL

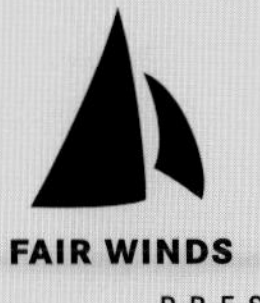

FAIR WINDS
PRESS

For my favorite boys in the world: Noah and Theo
May you dress well all your lives…
And for Hurtt
The world is less bright for your absence…

First published in the USA in 2006 by
Fair Winds Press, a member of
Quayside Publishing Group
33 Commercial Street
Gloucester, MA 01930

10 09 08 07 06 1 2 3 4 5

ISBN 1-59233-189-0

Library of Congress Cataloging-in-Publication Data
Neill, Emily.
Closet smarts : expert advice about : finding flattering fashions that don't cost a fortune, revamping your closet--what to keep, what to toss, what to wear with what, clothes you should never wear--and why, filling wardrobe gaps, the truth about color, clothes, and you / Emily Neill.
p. cm.
Includes index.
ISBN 1-59233-189-0
1. Clothing and dress. 2. Fashion. I. Title.
TT507.N36 2006
646'.34--dc22

2006010472

Cover design by Joan Lockhart
Book design by Carol Holtz of Holtz Design
Photography by Liz Linder of liz linder photography at www.lizlinder.com
Hair and makeup by Luiz Filho of LUZ Cosmetics at www.luzcosmetics.com
Clothing provided by LOOKS Boutique in Cambridge, Massachusetts

Printed and bound in China

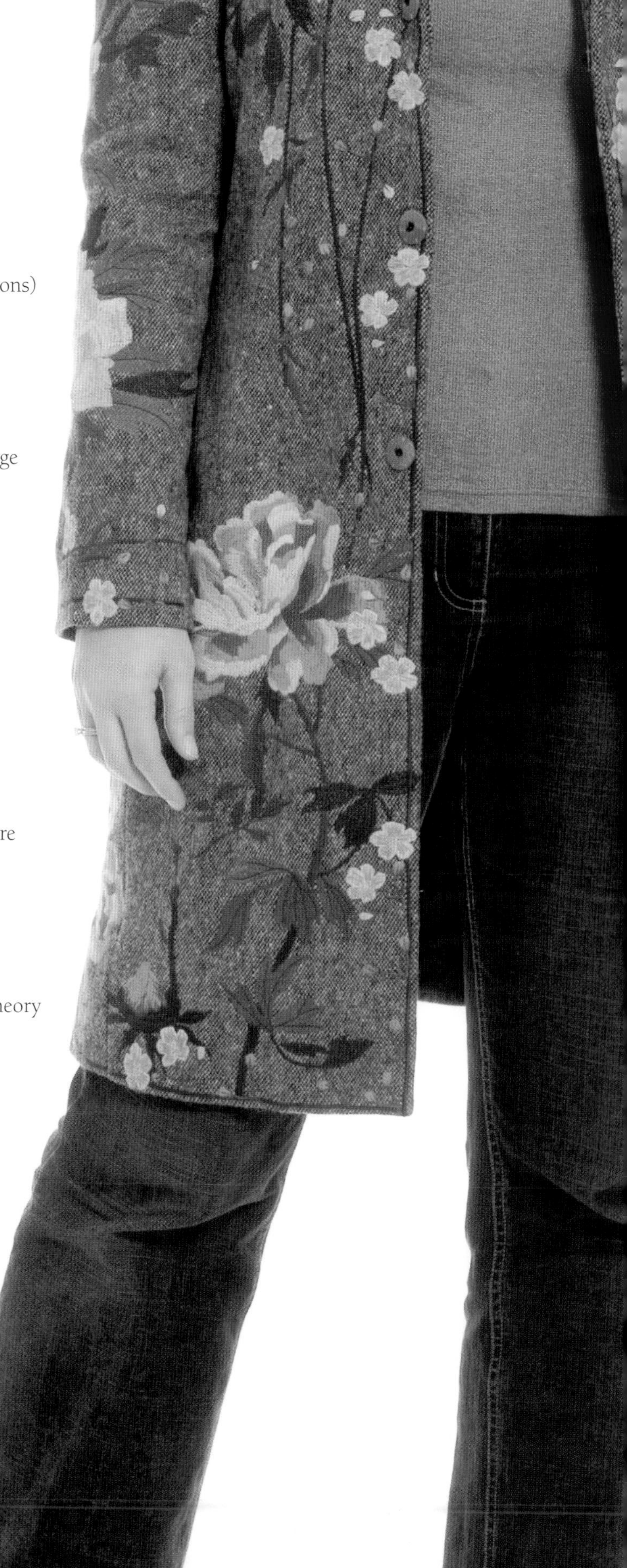

introduction

GETTING *YOUR* CLOSET SMARTS

We all know the feeling we get after reading fashion magazines, that combination of great hope and great shame. There is the great hope for what will be a new and better you *starting now*! And then, there is the great shame that comes when we look at the reality of our bodies in the mirror moments later—the love handles, back fat, sagging boobs, flabby arms, thunder thighs, cankles, knobby knees, or gangly limbs. The list of figure flaws is as endless as the stream of beautiful and seemingly perfect bodies we see marched out before us daily in magazines, TV shows, and movies and on billboards and the Internet.

Ultimately, the shock and dismay of looking at the reality of your body dissolves that feeling of sheer will you had mustered earlier that afternoon upon looking through your latest fashion mag. You recede into the indulgences of the every day—the demand for calories, regular life, and regular eating. You are left with the oh-so-*not* glamorous you, more likely to be found in jeans, a worn-out T-shirt, and clogs rather than heels, satin cargo pants, and a jeweled camisole. Why does it always feel so either/or, like if we can't look like what we see in a magazine, it isn't worth trying at all? How have our psyches trapped us into this shame spiral that sucks the life and glamour out of everyday living as most of us *really* live it? There is something terribly wrong with this zero-sum equation.

In my opinion, it is completely possible to look great in clothing whether you are a size 0 or a size 24, regardless of what you may think of the shape of your birthday suit underneath. This book is not about trying to talk you out of your firmly held belief that your thighs could smother a small elephant or that your shoulders could earn you a spot on the defensive line of the New England Patriots. I'll leave that to your therapist, your loyal friends, and even your partner, though I am doubtful that anyone can talk you out of your firmly held, body-hating ways. I am as guilty as you are, and I have no clue how to get those thoughts out of our collective body images, even after years of studying body politics.

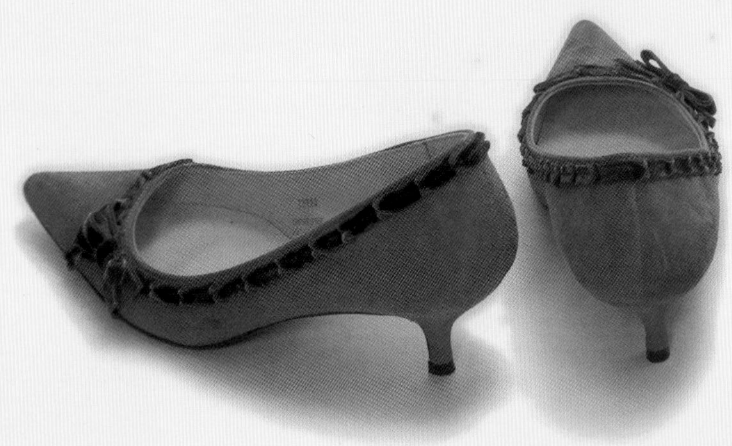

I *am* here to help, though, and I think I can. Because I am pretty darn sure I can bring glamour back into your everyday life, the kind that comes from knowing you look great, whatever your personal style, based on dressing better every day, in clothes that accentuate your best parts and mask the parts you'd like to take out back and shoot. I am talking about reintroducing you to that inner glow that comes usually just once a month or so, when you don your favorite outfit, the only thing in your closet you feel is fail-safe.

Why can't every day feel that way? Why can't we look great in all the clothes we have? Why must our wardrobes torture us rather than work for us? This book is dedicated to the inner glamourpuss in all of us, and it *won't* require getting back into those skinny jeans you are still saving from your college days. In fact, it will require that you once for all get *rid* of those psychological torture mechanisms called skinny clothes and learn to dress the body you live in. This is a skill any *body* can acquire, and the payoff is huger than you think your butt is. I promise.

In the chapters that follow, I hope to show you some basic fashion tricks that can sculpt your silhouette into the well-proportioned and shapely figure that you don't currently think you have. We all have *something* we like about our bodies, and even if it's your ears, I plan on showing you how to draw people's eyes to that spot and smooth over all the other rough spots.

I have personally been a clotheshorse for years. I grew up at the bottom of a four-person hand-me-down chain—all with very few funds for the most part—and I have always found a way. I have been a size two and a size sixteen, and I have borne two children, so I've gained quite a lot of first-hand closet smarts.

Over the years, I also started noticing that lots of women seemed to need help with their clothing choices. Many of them just seemed to throw on whatever came to hand first, while others had made an effort, but their choices only emphasized the figure flaws they were clearly trying to conceal. I couldn't just stand by and watch! So I started my business, Closet Smarts, and I have worked with hundreds of women—of all ages, shapes, sizes, and walks of life—to help them achieve a fashionable and eye-friendly figure. I hope you will find what follows to be as helpful as having me come over to your house and go through your closet with you, up close and personal. So take a deep breath and turn the page. You're that much closer to arriving at the best possible version of you!

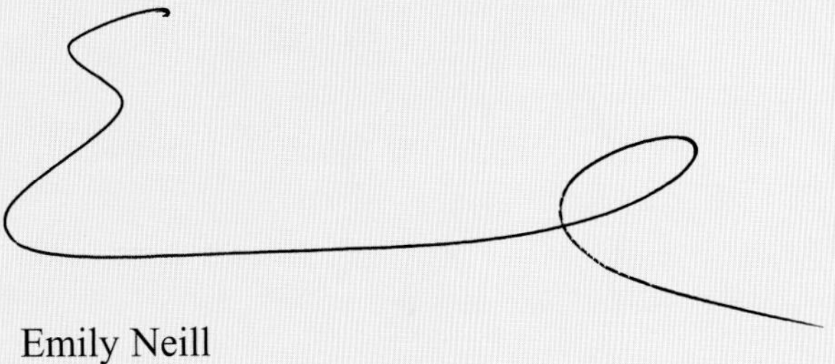

Emily Neill

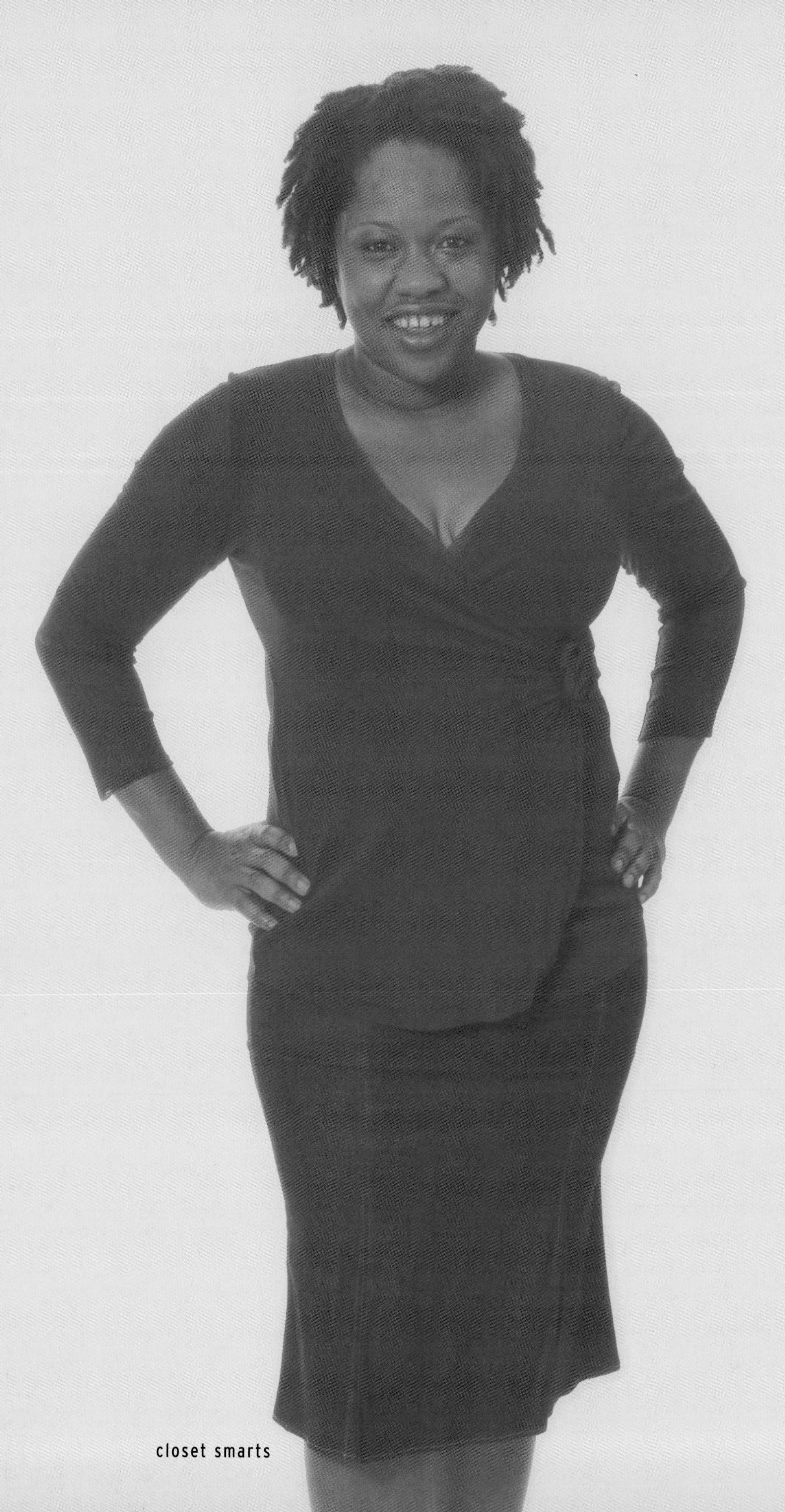

CHAPTER ONE

the myths we cling to

(Like Static on Nylons)

In this chapter, I'd like to introduce you to some of the basic fashion myths that plague most of us—consciously or unconsciously—and tend to keep us focused and stuck on our bodies as the source of "the problem." My philosophy, as someone who has worked with people of all shapes and sizes with their own wardrobes, is that there is a way for every body to look great in clothes; it's just a matter of finding the styles and cuts that really work for you. No problem! In this chapter, you'll meet ten lovely ladies of all shapes and sizes who will help you visualize certain figure challenges. Throughout the rest of the book, you can follow these gals through our style journey, and they will help show you the dos and don'ts that most closely mirror your own figure challenges.

Body Shapes: Breaking All the Rules

Let me guess. According to the experts and based on the choices of silhouette you've been given, you're a pear. Am I right? If I had a dime for every pear I've talked out of her tree, I could retire right now. It seems inevitable with the biologies we've been given that at some point along the path of our lives, things gravitate downward and outward, settling at or around Middle Earth. They hover there, increasing or decreasing an inch or two, but sadly, they slowly and inevitably distort our formerly better-proportioned bodies into Tweedledees and Tweedledums to varying degrees.

But our middle sections are only one small (well...) part of our overall silhouettes, and though the pear type may only very basically suggest that our tops are smaller than our middles, does this description really accurately capture the degree of variety that can take place on either side of our girths? Have you ever seen a fashion guide break the pear category into a typology of Bartletts, Boscs, and Anjous? Well, really, if they expect us to follow their golden rules of the fruit, they should be more specific, or at the very least give us a few more options for categorizing ourselves as we set out to readjust our wardrobes to accommodate our fruity centers.

Although plenty of fashion books have cut their teeth on quantifying a specific set of body types that should guide all fashion choices—the apple, the pear, the athletic build, the hourglass, etc.—I have found that bodies rarely fit these norms. Instead, most of us are some combination thereof, and often to such differing degrees that following a specific set of rules that always apply to the shape we've been squeezed into can be misleading and very limiting. Although it's reassuring to believe that the fashion industry knows what's out there in terms of our body shapes, and that it in fact designs for, or at the very least knows how to accommodate, these shapes, the reality isn't that simple. What designing for this list of silhouettes really does is to establish norms that we must all approximate.

THE TRUTH ABOUT BODY TYPES

Though I don't plan to spend this book exploding myths, I think there is a part of each of us that already knows this spiel from experience: On a very basic level, we just don't often see ourselves (i.e. our body shapes) represented anywhere in a realistic way where clothing is advertised or pictured.

Where we *do* see closer approximations of ourselves are in the special sections of fashion exposés, where suddenly the industry decides it has a conscience and maybe it should pretend to address the lion's share of *real* bodies that are actually trying to follow its designs and trends. Sadly, even within these special segments, where the average woman is apparently represented and her figure problems addressed, most of us are left with only a vague idea of where we fit into a continuum that, at best, completely oversimplifies the reality of our many shapes. At worst, this kind of typing, even as it claims to represent us, only sets us up to feel inadequate all over again as we squeeze ourselves into these cookie-cutter silhouettes that don't really describe us individually at all.

Of course, it's *convenient* to use these prototypes: How would anyone, in a three-page fashion spread, truly address the real variety of bodies that populate their readership? But when this limited dogma is used *everywhere*, in every outlet where women may search to find figure solutions, it gives the impression that these types are indeed real and true, and the reality of their convenience as a shorthand device slips out of our awareness.

From my perspective, as someone who works with real women on a daily basis as they struggle to dress their unique shapes fashionably, the psychology of these typologies does them—and almost certainly does *you*—an enormous disservice. Rather than helping real women find good advice about how to dress, these types seem more likely to hamper such efforts and distort women's ideas of themselves (as if we need any more help in this department!). Is it not enough that we are bombarded every day with images of women who are taller, thinner, and prettier than ourselves (usually through unnatural enhancement or distortion)?

REAL HELP FOR REAL BODIES

Must it be that even when we are (apparently) the subject of address, we end up with more of the same in a different guise? We need *real* help, and for me, real help comes in the form of a much larger variety of shapes than the fashion industry and its critical writers would have us shoehorn ourselves into.

In my line of work, where I deal with women of all shapes, sizes, ages, and lines of work, with all kinds of different phobias about their various body parts, my goal is always to work with each individual's unique shape. Although clearly, if you've picked up this book, you're hoping to find good advice—to tap into my expertise and get fashion help—help does not imply helplessness! My goal is to help each of you learn the fashion skills you need to help yourself.

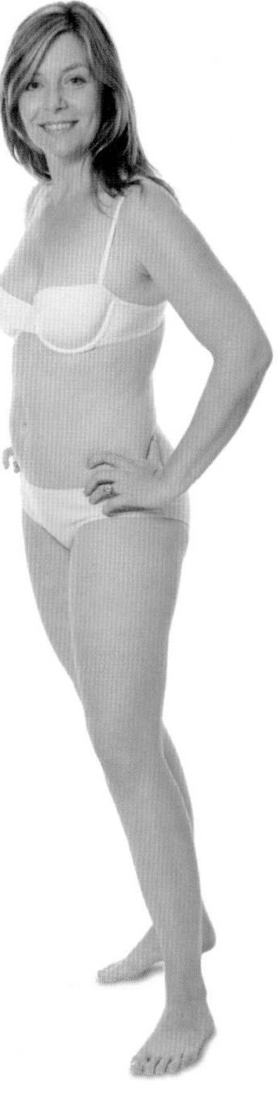

You've all heard the saying that if you give a man a fish, he'll eat for a day, but if you teach a man to fish, he'll eat for the rest of his life? Well, in my business, I always try to teach my clients to fish, rather than just feeding them the fashion industry line at the end of a hook. While the fashion industry's survival depends on creating an endless need for its (often contradictory) advice, I'd really like to teach you how *not* to need me... though I hope you will always enjoy reading my books.

FORGET THE STEREOTYPES —LOOK AT THE CLOTHES!

I'm going to start by assuming that you're an intelligent woman who wants to be involved in your own fashion choices—that you're capable of taking the principles of fashion, style, design, and basic silhouette I'll give you here and applying them to yourself, your own unique body. You with me?

Rather than starting out by telling you there are a few types of bodies, yours is one of them, and here is your set of fashion rules to never, ever veer from for time immemorial, I prefer to break down the body by those categories of clothing we typically wear as a starting point. Why? First of all, because there are far fewer styles and cuts of clothing to choose from than there are body types—at least from where I sit writing to you all out there. My idea is, rather than artificially trying to squeeze all of you into a few silhouettes and base my advice on the assumption that you fit one of these molds, why not focus on the *real* problem area: ill-fitting clothes?

This brings to mind a cartoon I once saw posted in the dressing room of a clothing store. It was entitled "Common Figure Flaws," and there were three silhouettes drawn. The first was called "pear shape," the second "short waist," and the third was a silhouette of a woman with a very unusually shaped head with the caption "poorly drawn head." Exactly! We have spent enough of our time obsessing about our apparent figure flaws.

Now, let's take a look at what's wrong with those clothes. Another reason I take this approach is because it in many ways more closely mirrors how we each actually approach our bodies when we get dressed every morning: We open our closets and drawers, and we pick, basically, a top and a bottom, right? Within those confines, there are further variations. We can pick *types* of tops—camisoles, blouses, sweaters, or turtlenecks (heaven forbid!), with different necklines and shapes—horseshoe, V-neck, scoopneck, boatneck, empire, box cut, shirred, or ruched.

The same goes for our bottoms and dresses. We can choose dresses, skirts, pants, or capris, and they can vary by shape and cut—pleated, low-waisted, boot-cut, straight-leg, A-line, bias cut, knee length, mid-calf, etc. What we have to learn, then, is *which* cuts look good on *our* figures. This is pretty obvious, I know. How we will go about determining this, however, *is* new and will hopefully leave you feeling addressed and better dressed, rather than once again misrepresented and misunderstood.

1

Body Transformations: What Clothes Can't Do

Another myth set out before the style-hungry (that would be us) that is shamelessly promoted by such shows as *The Swan* and *The Biggest Loser* is the notion that your *actual body* will somehow be transformed given the right clothes. The flip side of this immediate-gratification mindset is the one that repeatedly defeats us as we set out to deal with the reality of the bodies we have been given—that ongoing mantra that we will put off investing in our wardrobes and ourselves until we have lost those elusive five or ten pounds.

I have had clients who put off feeling good about themselves for *years* as they have battled back and forth across the line of some magic number that gets them off their self-punishing hook and makes them acceptable to themselves. I can't say how we get these hooks in us (though I certainly have my theories) or why we hang ourselves from them so relentlessly. What I *can* say is, they are never a reason to put off looking good and feeling good, *right now*. It's possible, and the results for your life and your head let alone your waistline are immeasurable. I hope that is why you picked up this book.

WHAT CLOTHES CAN DO FOR YOU

The reality is, with the right clothes, you can change the silhouette of your body, and this is key to the ideas presented in this book. My goal in guiding you to the right clothes choices is to help you *create a shape*, one you can accept, and, hopefully, one you can embrace and be proud of. I will help you create your best shape by making you look slimmer, helping you to create or show off well-proportioned curves, elongating your silhouette, accentuating your best assets, drawing the eye to those most universally attractive parts of a woman's body and *away* from trouble spots. I'll also show you how to give the overall appearance of being put together, purposeful, and stylish in your look, and thus confident and appealing.

Looking good and shapely in the clothes you wear goes a long way toward boosting your self-esteem in many departments. I see it every day in my line of work. But let's not kid ourselves. Underneath it all, unless we are eating sensibly and exercising enough to burn off more calories than we eat, we are going to find ourselves inhabiting the same bodies at the end of the day. Whether we love or hate our bodies in

Why not focus on the real problem area—ill-fitting clothes?

all their nakedness is a very loaded issue, and one particularly poignant for women in our culture. I don't propose to solve your body issues, but I *do* want to give you the tools to address them through clothing, which, though superficial, can go a long way toward transforming your outward appearance.

I strongly believe that this kind of outward transformation often gives women the motivation to make changes in their lives that lead them to gradually accept themselves and their bodies for what they are. Though my views are perhaps a reversal from the age-old adage that one should start from the inside when cultivating self-love and acceptance, I've seen with my own eyes the kind of transformation great outfits and wardrobes can inspire in the women who invest in them, and it is *not* a superficial investment.

With the right clothes, you can change your silhouette and create your own shape.

Body Image: Where Do We Go from Here?

To sum up, I don't expect to transform your body image, much as I'd like to convince you that your butt isn't really flat and your arms are perfectly normal-sized. I think it's ridiculous for someone who has never met you and has no idea about the clothes you've struggled to look good in to just announce, "You are *not fat*!" and expect that—poof!—you'll magically get over your body hatreds. I am not that naïve, my friend:

I know your issues with your shoulders and butt and ankles are far deeper-rooted than that.

So given these imperfections—imagined, distorted, or grounded in reality—where do we start? If you indeed have heavy arms and hate them and feel like you want to cover them all the time, and some fashion rule book says that if you've got heavy arms, you should never ever don short sleeves, much less contemplate—gasp!—going sleeveless, where does that really leave you? What about summer? Are you truly convinced that you can never bare your arms unless they're trim and toned?

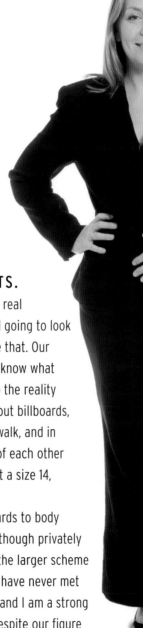

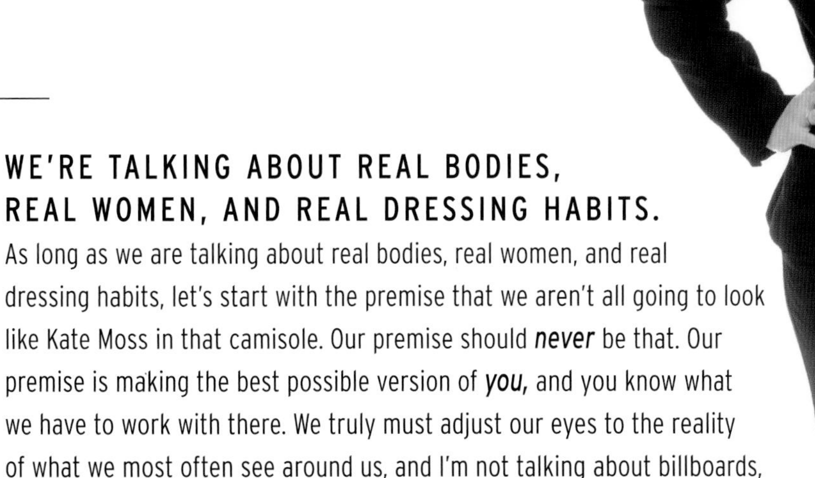

WE'RE TALKING ABOUT REAL BODIES, REAL WOMEN, AND REAL DRESSING HABITS.

As long as we are talking about real bodies, real women, and real dressing habits, let's start with the premise that we aren't all going to look like Kate Moss in that camisole. Our premise should ***never*** be that. Our premise is making the best possible version of ***you,*** and you know what we have to work with there. We truly must adjust our eyes to the reality of what we most often see around us, and I'm not talking about billboards, TV, and magazines. I'm talking about on the bus, on the sidewalk, and in the cubicle next to you. Women may be the harshest critics of each other and of themselves, but nonetheless, most women are at least a size 14, and no taller than 5'4".

That is all the preaching I am going to do here with regards to body image. But I am here to say that what you see in the mirror, though privately terrifying and terrible to you each and every morning, is, in the larger scheme of things, probably pretty average, and ***certainly*** workable. I have never met a body I could not work with (read: improve) in all my years, and I am a strong believer that with a little tweaking and training of the eye, despite our figure flaws, we can still look pretty good amongst our peers—and in fact, ***that*** should be our goal. The key? Choosing the right version of a particular cut to flatter your best parts and obscure the rest.

MAKING THE MOST OF YOUR ASS(ETS)

Essential to getting to that best possible version of you is homing in on your best assets and maximizing their attention-grabbing potential in any outfit or ensemble. Though, as I said earlier, I won't try to convince you in this book to dispense with your negative bodily obsessions, I *would* like to convince you that there are beautiful parts of you. And I bet you know what they are. What's more, I'd love to teach you how to make yourself feel like those are the parts of you that are always making a first impression. It's actually one of the simplest principles we will work on throughout this book.

So if you want to start now, think "nice butt," "toned arms," "slim ankles," "great breasts," and keep those thoughts foremost in your mind; we will find a way to work it, I promise. If you're having trouble, I can tell you this without even meeting you: For the most part, a woman's décolletage (the area below her neck and above her breasts) is a great focal point for any outfit, and it should never be obscured if at all possible. The cut of a great top is one of the key ways to draw the eye where most women want it—up and away from hips, thighs, bellies, and butts—i.e., as far away from Middle Earth or Tweedledee/dum territory as possible.

Throughout the chapters that follow, as we work our way through the average wardrobe, such tips as opening up the décolletage will be a primary focus for teaching you how to work your assets and how to obscure your trouble spots. A key aspect of this strategy will be teaching you how to build a well-proportioned silhouette. Imagine yourself now, in a photo, with callouts pointing out all the successful elements of your truly put-together look. This *will* be you, I promise.

Real Fashion versus High Fashion

I am going to tell you right now, whether you consider it a confession of inadequacy or a badge of honor, I am a reality-based fashionista. From where I stand, even if you need help with fashion, I bet that you are already a lot more reality-based about dressing than most folks in the fashion industry are. Don't believe it? Read on, and you'll soon see yourself.

You shop at the most popular mall stores, big discount department stores, and high-end retailers. You get a million catalogs and loyally flip through all of them, folding down the pages of items you will order someday to fill out your imagined perfect wardrobe and returning the catalogs to the pile next to your bed to collect dust indefinitely (or until you get the next one). You keep your underwear for too long, and you have stockings that you've had for three years with runs that start above where your skirt does or on the bottom of the footie part (so why not keep them?).

You put your bras in the dryer, and they have pills. You have blouses with sweat stains under the arms and probably a few pairs of pants with pleats and maybe even tapered legs. You have one winter coat that you've had for *at least* the past two seasons. You have no more than ten pairs of shoes, and you wear them all (into the ground, no doubt), even when they don't make you feel so great about how you look. You probably even wear sneakers on your commute in to work, don't you?

And you have no idea, really, about the overall impact of your "outfit," because you probably don't have a full-length mirror in your house in which you might be able to see (and assess) your entire ensemble. If you are at all interested in checking out how you look, you probably stand on your toilet to use your bathroom vanity mirror (conveniently overlooking the issue of your shoes).

Not that there's anything wrong with that. It's just that, as you know since you picked up this book, you could probably do better. You could be more deliberate about what you buy, and you could replace just about everything you own, soon, and you could actually look really great, all the time, not just when it's your favorite outfit's turn in the fashion rotation.

Tell me this isn't you, or hasn't been you at some time in the recent past? This is called reality, my friend, and there wouldn't be such a thing as rose-colored glasses if reality didn't get ugly sometimes, or at the very least, mundane and in need of a silver lining, or how about a silver metallic pair of kitten heels? Anyone? Anyone?

So, what's my message to you as a reality-based fashionista? What I'm trying to tell you is, do not *fear* me. I am not a monster or some disenchanted ex-fashion guru tossed from the runways of Milan and ready to pretend I know your plight as the "average woman" and what you're all about. In fact, I am as reality-based as you are. I shop where you shop, have my fair share of horror in the dressing room, work within a budget, contract and expand through the years and seasons, hate my arms... the list goes on.

I'm your friendly neighborhood fashionista, facing the struggles you struggle with, and I know how you think. I also know what you are after, if you only had the time, or the know-how, or the consistent energy to apply in this department. That's what I do for people as a living, and that's what I am prepared to do for you here, in a language and with examples that you can actually find "out there"—and maybe even on sale!

The Truth about Color

What about color? Here is another topic fashion experts are eager to give advice about—cookie-cutter advice, as far as I'm concerned. You often hear things like "black is flattering on *everyone*," and "brown is the new black!" If we followed what fashion magazines had to say about color, we would be tossing our wardrobes every other season.

Then there is the cult of "color me beautiful." You know the one, the seasonal approach to color science. Who are these people who divide up the world of color into four seasons and make us choose only *one*? Why are we so ready to cut out a whole range of colors from our fashion choices simply to fit into a cookie-cutter prescription for avoiding fashion mistakes? "Color me beautiful" is the Atkins diet approach to color. It seems simple when you start out, an easy answer to some of your most anxious self-image problems. And yet there seems to be something eerily wrong with its prescriptions as you cling to its rules. When all you eat is meat and cheese, or all you feel safe wearing are cool blues and greens, you know that can't be the full story. And I'm here to tell you, it's not.

In my business, I always ask clients the questions, "Are there colors you consider out of your range?" and then, "Have you ever rediscovered a color you thought wasn't 'you' in the past?" Inevitably, the first list is long, and there is always at least one color that pops up in the reclaimed category. How did we get here? I'll tell you how: It's because we were told over and over again that there are colors we can and cannot wear, and we bought it hook, line, and sinker.

I absolutely disagree with this methodology of color, and I'll tell you why. Because color is so dynamic and varied—in terms of shade, hue, depth, and texture—that any absolute statement about any color is never always true—for *anyone*. There is such a huge range of color out there, so many *different* reds and oranges and blues, not to mention the gradations from white to cream, that to rule out any color before you go into the dressing room seems an unnecessary limitation.

I will show you in the pictures that follow what I believe simply isn't true—that whole families of color are off limits to certain people. I cannot stress this enough as you start experimenting a little with your fashion excursions, because who *hasn't* had the experience of putting something on they normally would not and seeing a whole new side of themselves? This should tell us something.

Sure, there are colors that look *better* on us than others, but don't eliminate any color as you shop. Even if you are not a big fan of shopping and don't consider it a fun or playful activity, we all must do it. As you wander around the racks to choose a handful of try-ons, try not to discriminate based on color. In fact, if you are going to take risks with anything typically out of your bounds, *start* with color. I promise you, you will see with your own eyes how much wiggle room there truly is when it comes to color.

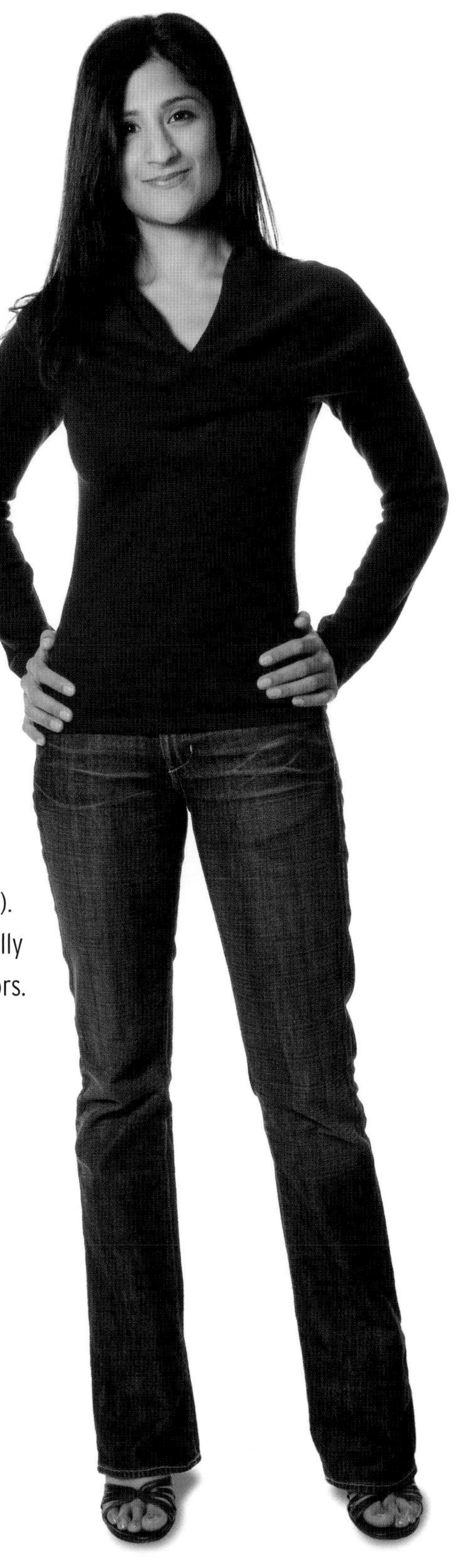

AVOID PRIMARY COLORS.

I have to give one piece of advice as you begin to branch out: Avoid primary colors (straight-up blues, yellows, and reds) and look for muted hues and heathered fabrics (those with several blended hues of the same color or mixes of gray or black with another color). Primary colors have no subtlety whatsoever, and unless you are really going for a deliberately splashy look, they don't do anyone any favors. Look for olives, plums, smoky blues, wine reds, and mocha browns. This type of color family, known as neutrals, tend to blend better with each other to expand your wardrobe's mixing and matching possibilities. They are also more adaptable to different skin types and hair colors, and they are more sophisticated in tone for your overall self-presentation.

The False Comfort of Rules: An Alternative

The fashion business seems to thrive on people's fears and insecurities, and what that leads most fashion writers to do is make up some easy list of ten rules to follow for a fail-safe method of dressing. But why should dressing well be any different than any other challenge we have anxiety about in our lives? My drift: If it sounds too good to be true, it probably is. Is what we all really want just a set of ten rules to follow that will always and forever be true? What happens, then, when our bodies change? When we become mothers (or hit thirty) and everything shifts around? Or our careers change, or even our priorities, all of which may provoke shifts in our dressing habits, needs, and desires?

If the rules approach was truly effective, fashion magazines would be out of business.

I am going to assume that you have started to get a sinking feeling with regards to these lists of rules when it comes to getting answers and workable solutions to your particular fashion problems. If the rules approach was truly effective, fashion magazines would be out of business, because everyone would already know everything they needed to know about how to dress as well as the fashion experts do. I am not a fan of rules, and I will try hard not to present any of my fashion insights in this book in the form of rules to be followed.

When pressed to come up with a short quip about fashion dos and don'ts, I swear the only thing I can say with certainty is that pleats are flattering on no one's midsection, and that tapered pants don't do anyone's silhouette any favors. But I swear, that's it. The rest is experiment and play, assessing the individual and creating proportion on that particular body through clothing structure and design. It's different for *every* body, and that is why I eschew subscribing either to archetypal body types or rules as a way of training your eye to make the best choices for your particular shape.

The most honest and helpful way for me to teach you how to achieve the best possible version of you, is by showing you as many different kinds of bodies as I can and letting you mix and match your parts and apply the tricks of design that I demonstrate for you. You may luck out and find that a particular model in this book matches your proportions almost exactly. But what is more likely is that there will be *parts* of all the women shown here that reflect *parts* of you.

This is reality, and the good news is, it's totally workable! I wouldn't bother to write this book with the premise of redressing the methodologies of other fashion-advice books if I didn't think the dressing public needed to see this, presented *this way*, rather than as it has traditionally been discussed and presented. And so, let us begin, again, anew, without presuppositions. Forget what you thought you knew about your shape, about rules of any kind, about fashion dos and don'ts.

Just let it go and take a deep breath. I am about to introduce you to ten very real bodies, women just like yourselves, who come in all different shapes and sizes, from all walks of life. They will revisit you throughout these chapters as we work our way through the basics of dressing well every day. I am not going to organize them into discrete categories, because I believe every body is unique, and as such presents unique challenges. In what follows, I will let you know how these women see their bodies and their particular fashion challenges and how I see them.

Throughout the rest of the book, we will work on how these gals dress themselves, and I'll show you (and them) how they might dress themselves to better enhance their figures. Again, you may not resemble any one of these women, but the way I will work with their bodies throughout the book will give you the chance to identify which *parts* of them most closely resemble your own parts, and you can mix and match my fashion advice to suit you. So without further ado, here they are!

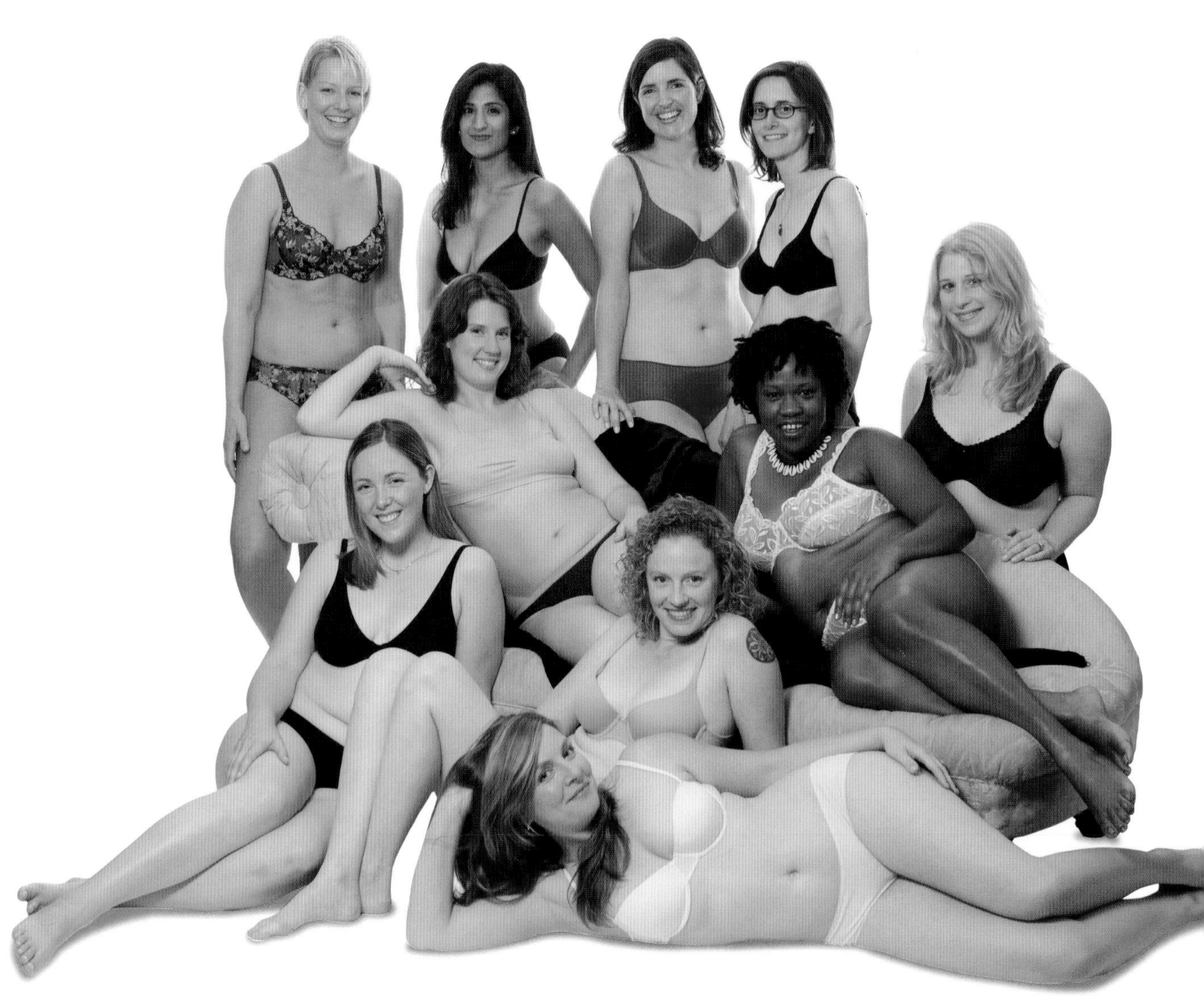

1

a gallery of body types

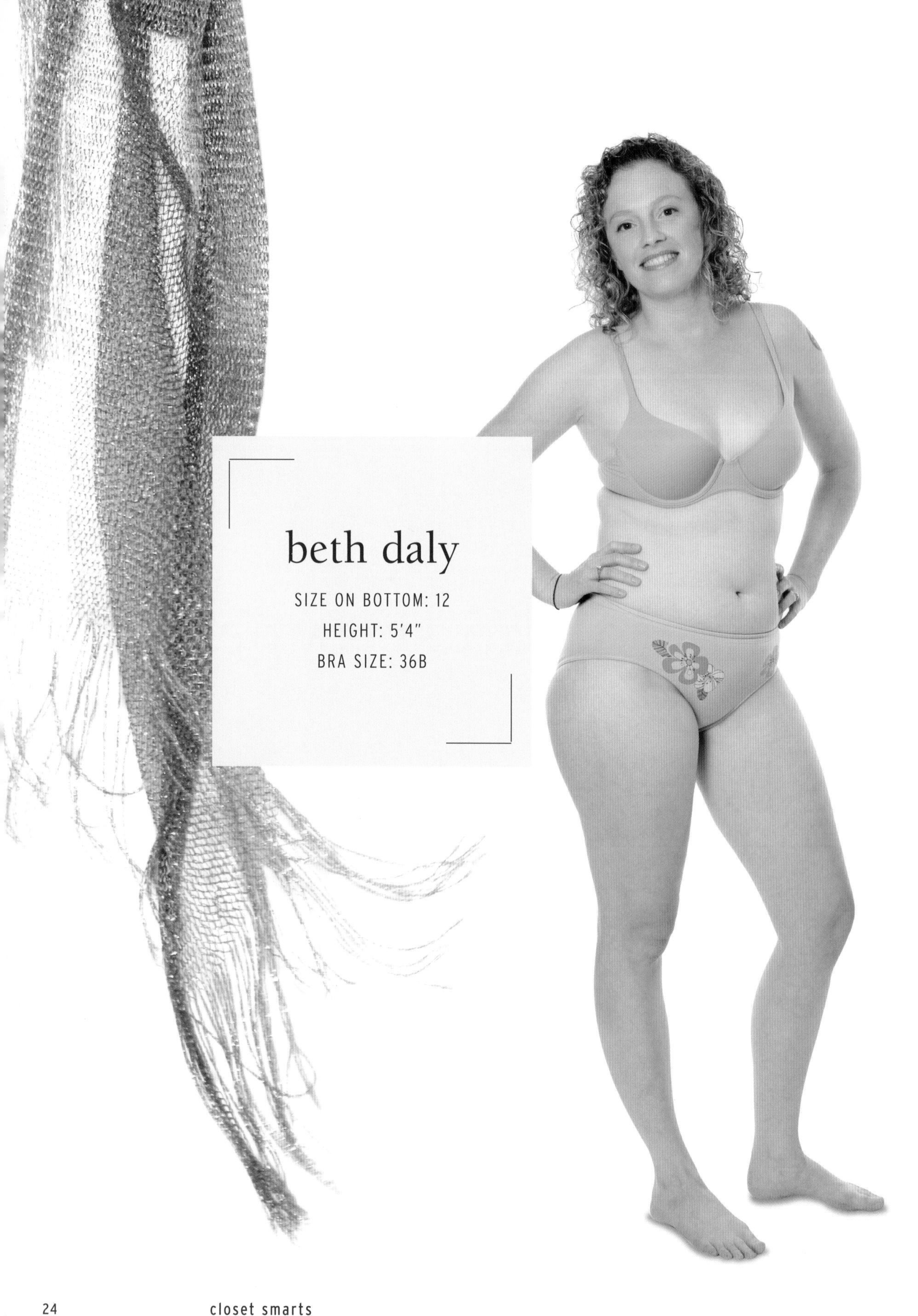

beth daly

SIZE ON BOTTOM: 12

HEIGHT: 5'4"

BRA SIZE: 36B

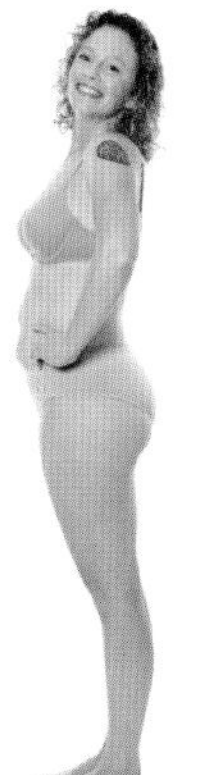 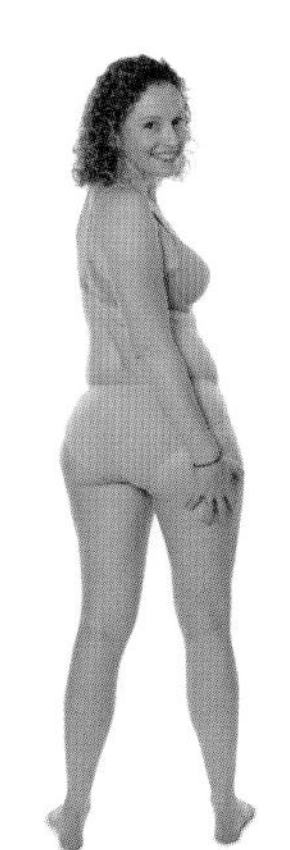 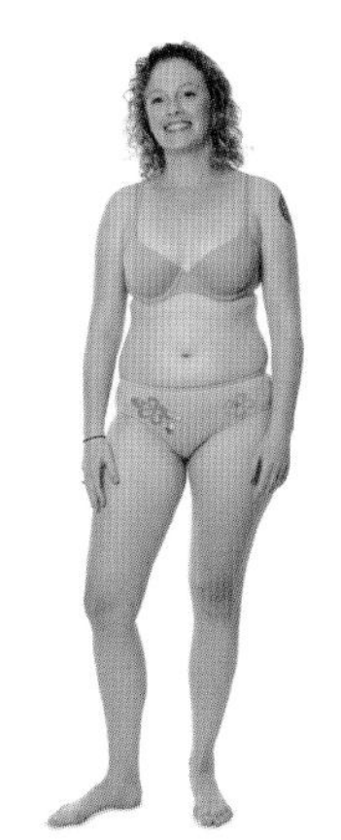 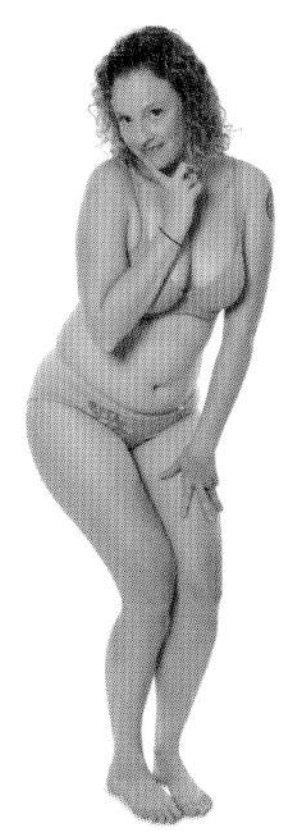 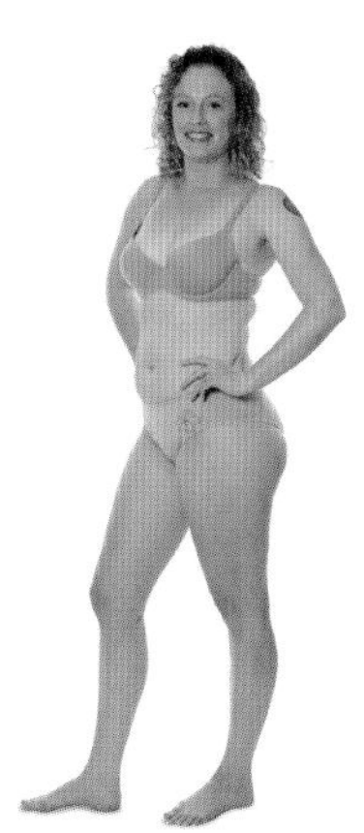

1

she says:

"When I get up in the morning and get dressed, my biggest 'body-part' challenge is my rear end and hips. Let's face it, I'm pear shaped. My top half is nice and small: narrow shoulders (which purses slip off of) and small arms and hands. Then we travel downward and move up an entire size! I find that dresses are often too big on top, too tight on the bottom. Thank God for A-lines, otherwise I'd never wear a dress. When it comes to pants, I get very frustrated. The cute low-rise boot-cut does not look good on my womanly hips. Boot-cut pants tend to accent them instead of flatter them. My butt looks like a bubble! I tend to do best with straight-leg pants, with more room in the rear and the thighs. I don't want to feel like an old lady, though, having to wear older-people pants and cut off from the cute funky pants."

i say:

"Beth's woes are quite common. Most women are not proportionately shaped and are either larger on the top or bottom. (Larger on the bottom is more common.) With a mid-rise, straight-leg pant, Beth has a chance to even out her proportions, and her small top can carry a good layered look that simultaneously shows off her petite upper half, while adding some structure to balance out the proportion of her shoulders and hips. She is right that an A-line shape will work best on her for skirts and dresses. Choosing stiffer fabrics that will provide a good shape will help her avoid showing any bumps or lumps in her rear, thighs, and belly area."

felisha foster

SIZE ON TOP: 6

SIZE ON BOTTOM: 8-10

HEIGHT: 5'5"

BRA SIZE: 36B

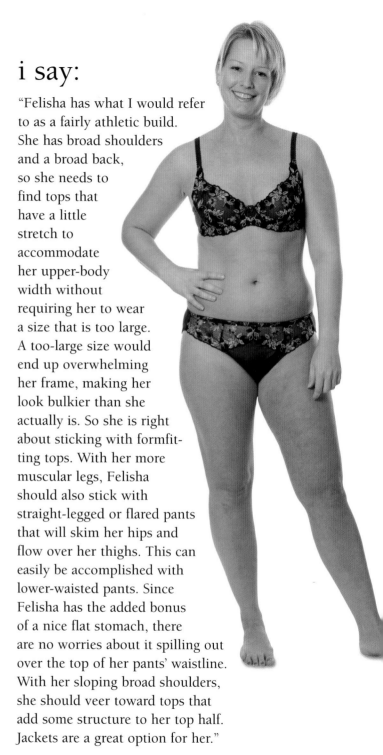

she says:

"Honestly, I struggle every morning when I look in the mirror to get dressed. I have always wanted to be taller and thinner. I cannot stand my legs so I never wear shorts. I have fairly large extremities, so sleeveless shirts are out as well. My stomach has always been the smallest part of my body so I try to accentuate it. I try to wear tops that are formfitting to give me a small look up top. Finding pants is a struggle, because I have fairly large legs. I wear boot-cut jeans and pants as well as long skirts to elongate my figure. I try to wear heels as much as possible to give the illusion that I am actually taller and thinner than I am."

i say:

"Felisha has what I would refer to as a fairly athletic build. She has broad shoulders and a broad back, so she needs to find tops that have a little stretch to accommodate her upper-body width without requiring her to wear a size that is too large. A too-large size would end up overwhelming her frame, making her look bulkier than she actually is. So she is right about sticking with formfitting tops. With her more muscular legs, Felisha should also stick with straight-legged or flared pants that will skim her hips and flow over her thighs. This can easily be accomplished with lower-waisted pants. Since Felisha has the added bonus of a nice flat stomach, there are no worries about it spilling out over the top of her pants' waistline. With her sloping broad shoulders, she should veer toward tops that add some structure to her top half. Jackets are a great option for her."

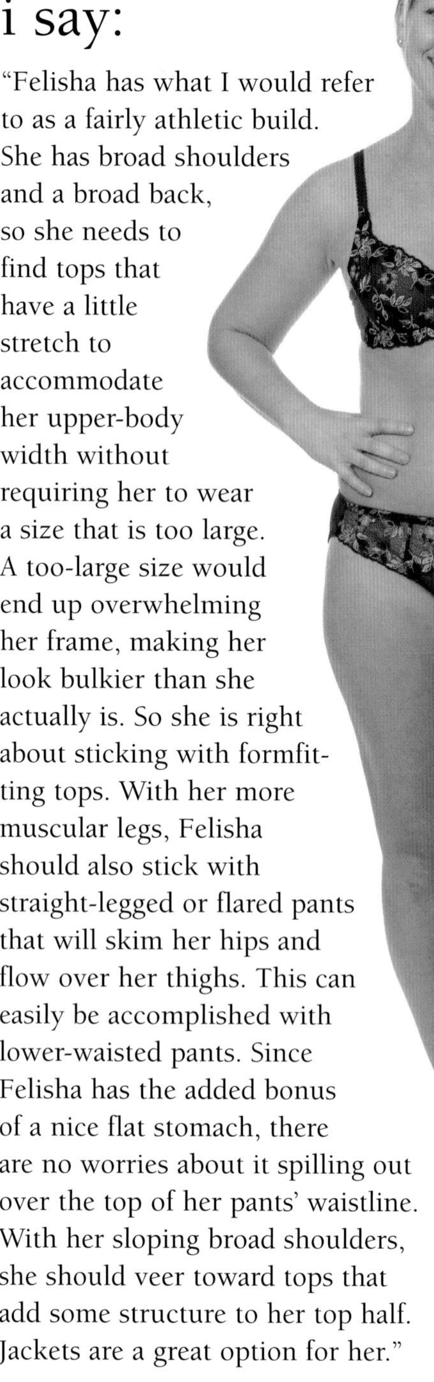

she says:

"When I look in the mirror before getting dressed, I think of my biggest figure challenge as my bulging stomach, which makes it impossible for me to wear tops tucked in with belts. I spend most of the day sucking it in! Also, I struggle with my wide shoulders and bigger upper body. I feel like I am top-heavy in most outfits, and I don't know how to pick the right tops."

sara wilkinson

SIZE ON TOP: 8-10

SIZE ON BOTTOM: 8

HEIGHT: 5'5"

BRA SIZE: 34C

i say:

"I can't say I agree with Sara that her biggest figure challenge is her 'bulging belly.' She's certainly better off than most of us. But she does have a very square shape, which is accentuated by her height and her broad shoulders. I see her most pressing figure challenge, then, as the need to soften up her shape, adding some curves and roundness to her shoulders in a way that would make her overall appearance more voluptuous and less boyish. She's got the hips and the height, and making sure her curves show through the waistline with higher-cut skirts and pants will help accentuate those hips in a good way. Adding some ruffle or poof around the shoulder line, or at least tops with softer lines (scoops, etc.), will also add to this softening illusion. Since she is taller than most, going for classic Hepburn lines in a wide-legged trouser and curve-hugging turtle-neck would really elongate her silhouette and show off all the curves she's got in their best possible light."

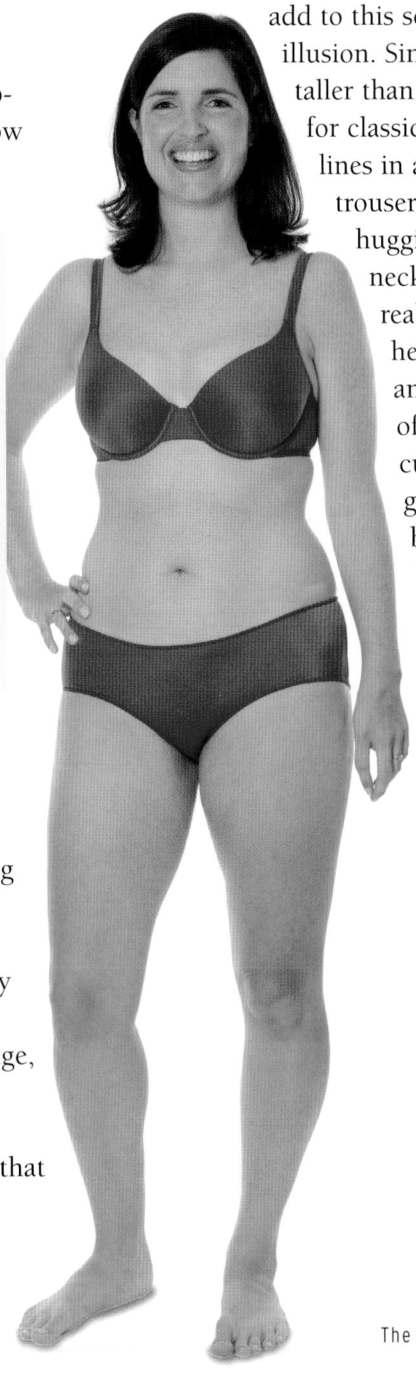

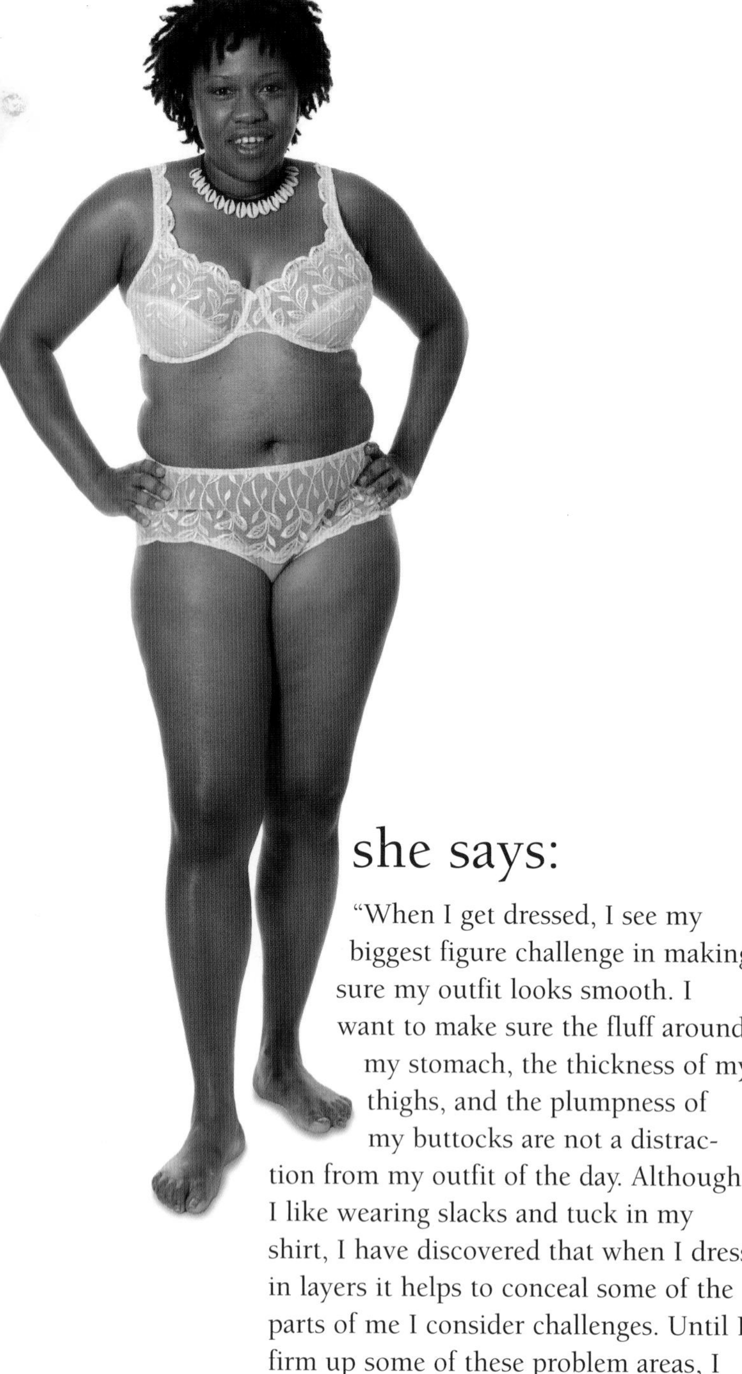

yvette wilkes

SIZE ON TOP: 12
(PETITE LARGE OR EXTRA-LARGE)
SIZE ON BOTTOM: 12-14
(PETITE LARGE OR EXTRA-LARGE)
HEIGHT: 5'2"
BRA SIZE: 38C

she says:

"When I get dressed, I see my biggest figure challenge in making sure my outfit looks smooth. I want to make sure the fluff around my stomach, the thickness of my thighs, and the plumpness of my buttocks are not a distraction from my outfit of the day. Although I like wearing slacks and tuck in my shirt, I have discovered that when I dress in layers it helps to conceal some of the parts of me I consider challenges. Until I firm up some of these problem areas, I always try to wear outfits that have at least two layers and to have a good slip for when I wear dresses without a jacket."

i say:

"Yvette may have a fuller figure, but she's got great shape. She needs to use her clothes to accentuate that shape, without either overdressing it with too many clothes of the boxy variety, or too few that hug her too tightly and accentuate girth rather than shapely curves. Suity looks with wider-legged pants and V-necks to draw attention to her face and neckline while minimizing her breasts are a great place to start. Stiffer fabrics will go a long way towards letting Yvette dress up her curves and her confidence without overexposing her challenging parts. Using styling details in her tops like ruching, princess seams, and wrap tops will also help mask her belly, while showing off other parts of her upper half, like her breasts and décolletage."

1

she says:

"Because my top and bottom (rack and back?) tend to take it for the team, I try to put together outfits that accentuate my middle, which so far has been spared despite the jiggle from my pregnancy. This means slim-fitting tops that hug my waist and lengthening wide-leg pants or longer skirts, in order to spread the whole effect vertically. I often try to simplify getting dressed by sticking to one top and one bottom, forgoing accessories and layers. This makes me bored with my clothes, and I feel as if I need more. I am always searching for the perfect top that does everything without me having to do more than pull it over my head. I love layers and the interest they provide—keeping the eye working. But when I try this, the effect is sometimes lost under the loose cardigans I choose. I love wrap tops or belting my waist, but I often forget to invest in accessories. I think by now I have plenty of clothes, but I am lazy and need ideas as to how to recombine them. I walk a lot and so avoid heels, but I love the height they offer, which elongates and straightens my curvy figure. However, the infinitely stylish and creative teachers at my son's preschool have inspired me with their utilitarian shoe choices, showing me that clogs and platforms can look great and do a good job of adding height. I try to incorporate them into my (hopefully) sophisticated and classic looks."

amy bebergal

SIZE ON TOP: SMALL

SIZE ON BOTTOM: 8

HEIGHT: 5'4"

BRA SIZE: 36C

i say:

"Amy is lucky to have a very proportionately shaped figure—what they call the classic hourglass. Her biggest figure challenge is thinning out 'the extras' (post-mommydom) and keeping the focus on that hourglass shape. She indeed has a waist, and I agree that it should be celebrated! Wearing clothes that are boxy or have too much material would be a great disservice, so she needs to focus on clothes that hug her figure without squeezing it and accentuating bulges. Heels would be a great accessory for her shorter stature, but the same effect can be achieved with the well-refined shape of a shoe, or even with just the smallest of heels."

karen santospago

SIZE ON TOP: MEDIUM (8-10)
SIZE ON BOTTOM: LARGE (12-14)
HEIGHT: 5'7"
BRA SIZE: 36C

she says:

"I think that my figure, while not petite, is in proportion, so I try to dress in proportion. My stomach is relatively flat. I carry most of my extra weight in my hips and thighs and upper arms.
I don't wear shorts ever. I will wear cropped pants that show off my ankles.
I don't wear shoes that make my feet look small. On the top, I often wear tailored three-quarter-sleeve tops with princess seams. This shows off my wrists and neck/chest, which are the thinnest parts of my figure."

i say:

"Karen has a very square shape that is determined in large part by a broad back. Lucky for her, as she quite rightly observes, her body is largely proportionate, so the trick for her in dressing is to choose clothes that create those extra elements of curve where she can (bust area, waistline, and hips). This will give her the appearance of a more hourglass-shaped silhouette, rather than a more boxy shape. She has the right idea in showing off the narrowest parts of her figure (ankles, wrists, and forearms), which will also draw attention away from the thicker parts of her figure and add to the illusion of being more fine-boned."

she says:

"My biggest challenge is that my waist is uneven because I have scoliosis. One side has a curvy shape and the other is straight. In addition, I have skinny legs and no butt. My solution is to wear pants or skirts that fall below my waist and wear my shirts out. One recent stroke of luck was that I can now get a lot of clothes I like in petite sizes. This is great because it saves me from having to get so many alterations!"

deborah wieder

SIZE ON TOP: EXTRA-SMALL

SIZE ON BOTTOM: PETITE 0-2

HEIGHT: 5'2"

BRA SIZE: 34B

i say:

"Deborah is your classic skinny Minnie. As she mentioned, besides having the challenge of finding clothes that don't completely overwhelm her frame, she has the added challenge of finding clothes that help give her a more even silhouette due to her scoliosis. In both cases, clothes with added structure and some girth will help create the shape that her figure lacks on its own merits. Structured jackets and thicker fabrics like wools and boucles as well as thicker cottons, denims, and even corduroys can help create this look. She can also carry bolder style elements like ruffles, layers, ribs, and textured prints, as long as they remain in proportion to her frame and not overwhelming. They will help mask the unevenness of her silhouette, while also adding some shape and curve to her narrow limbs. She should avoid clothes that draw attention to the skinniness of her limbs, which would have the effect of making her look scrawny rather than slender."

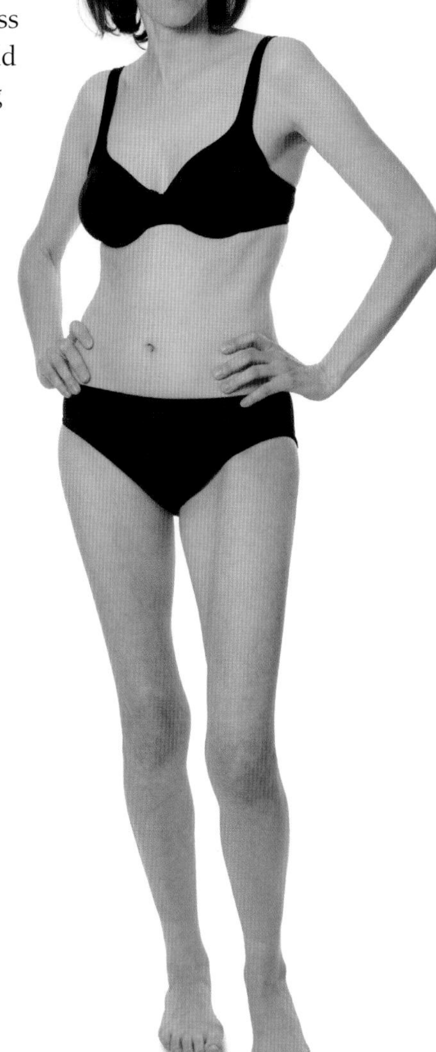

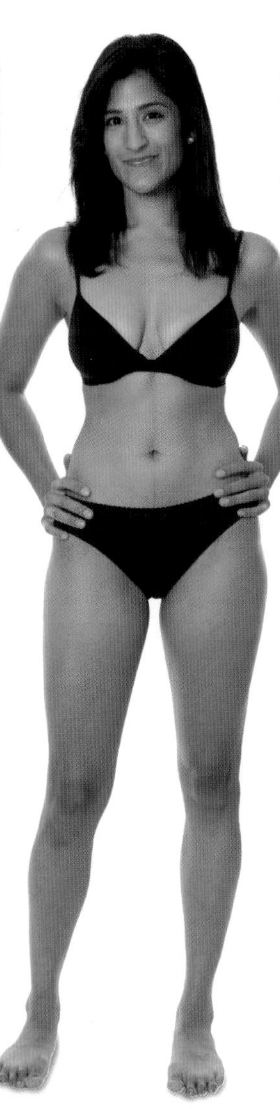

supriya mehta

SIZE ON TOP: 0-2

SIZE ON BOTTOM: 0-2

HEIGHT: 5'2 1/2"

BRA SIZE: 34B

she says:

"Although thin, I'm short-waisted and have relatively big boobs for my size Thus my goal when I dress is to elongate my torso (i.e., low-waisted everything and long tops), and I wear tops that do not draw attention to my disproportionately big boobs. If I'm being really critical, I could say I have a flat butt, though personally I'm not really looking for a JLo butt, just a firm one. My overall feeling is that while I look okay—I can put together an outfit for a date, meeting at work, presentation, etc.—85 percent of the time I don't look like I've dressed with a purpose in mind. Within that 85 percent, 10 percent of the time my clothes are boring, and an additional 15 percent of the time I come out looking dorky. Overall, as I struggle to work with my figure challenges, I tend to miss the overarching 'sass' factor."

i say:

"Supriya has the kind of figure you are probably all ogling right now, thinking how can there be anything wrong with that?!? But it's all relative, really. Any way you slice it, clothes can look bad (you'll see what I mean in the pages that follow). Supriya is not especially curvy outside the boob area, so she should be looking to create more of an hourglass shape with the use of styling details like cinched, cropped jackets, bias-cut (read hip-emphasizing) skirts, and fuller pant cuts. With her short waist, Supriya could really benefit by using the layering strategy, using longer shirts and shorter sweaters and jackets to elongate the silhouette of her waist. Because she is slender, she could also stand to add a little girth and shape through the structure of her clothes. This may be best achieved through structured mini-jackets, bulkier knit sweaters, wider-legged pants, and fuller-cut skirts. She should steer away from clothes that really cling to her and make her arms and legs look scrawny or emphasize her large bust, creating a disproportionate top half."

she says:

"When I look in the mirror before getting dressed, I think of my biggest figure challenges as my thighs. I grew up in a multicultural neighborhood, where a round butt and thick thighs were a good thing. But as I've gotten older, I feel pressured to have skinny thighs like all the models and celebrities I see in fashion magazines. Sometimes I think if they were just a little firmer, I wouldn't care that they were thick. After all, I think a strong athletic body is very sexy. But it's the softness and the not-so-smooth cellulite that bothers me. All the rest I don't mind so much. I know I have wide hips and a round butt, but like I said, I grew up thinking that wasn't a bad thing. Of course, there are the bad days (hello, PMS!) when I think that I look greatly disproportionate, that my boobs are too small, my butt is too big, that I have knobby knees..."

i say:

"Morgan is blessed with one of the best assets for anyone with thick anything, height! She has a good start in working on creating a well-proportioned silhouette. What she needs to look out for is wearing items that cut her at her widest parts, the hips, butt, and thigh area. Her best friends in this department will be longer skirts that sweep off of her hips, straighter-legged and wide-cuffed pants that also brush off her hips and create proportion at the bottom of her silhouette, and tops that draw attention to her waistline or rib cage (her narrowest parts) as a focal point."

morgan stockmayer

SIZE ON TOP: 10-12

SIZE ON BOTTOM: 10-12 SKIRTS, 12-14 PANTS

HEIGHT: 5'11"

BRA SIZE: 34C

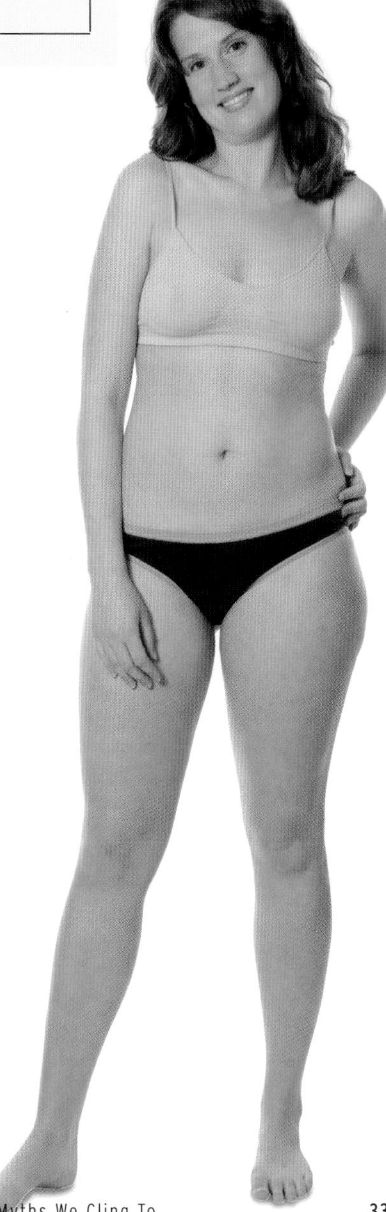

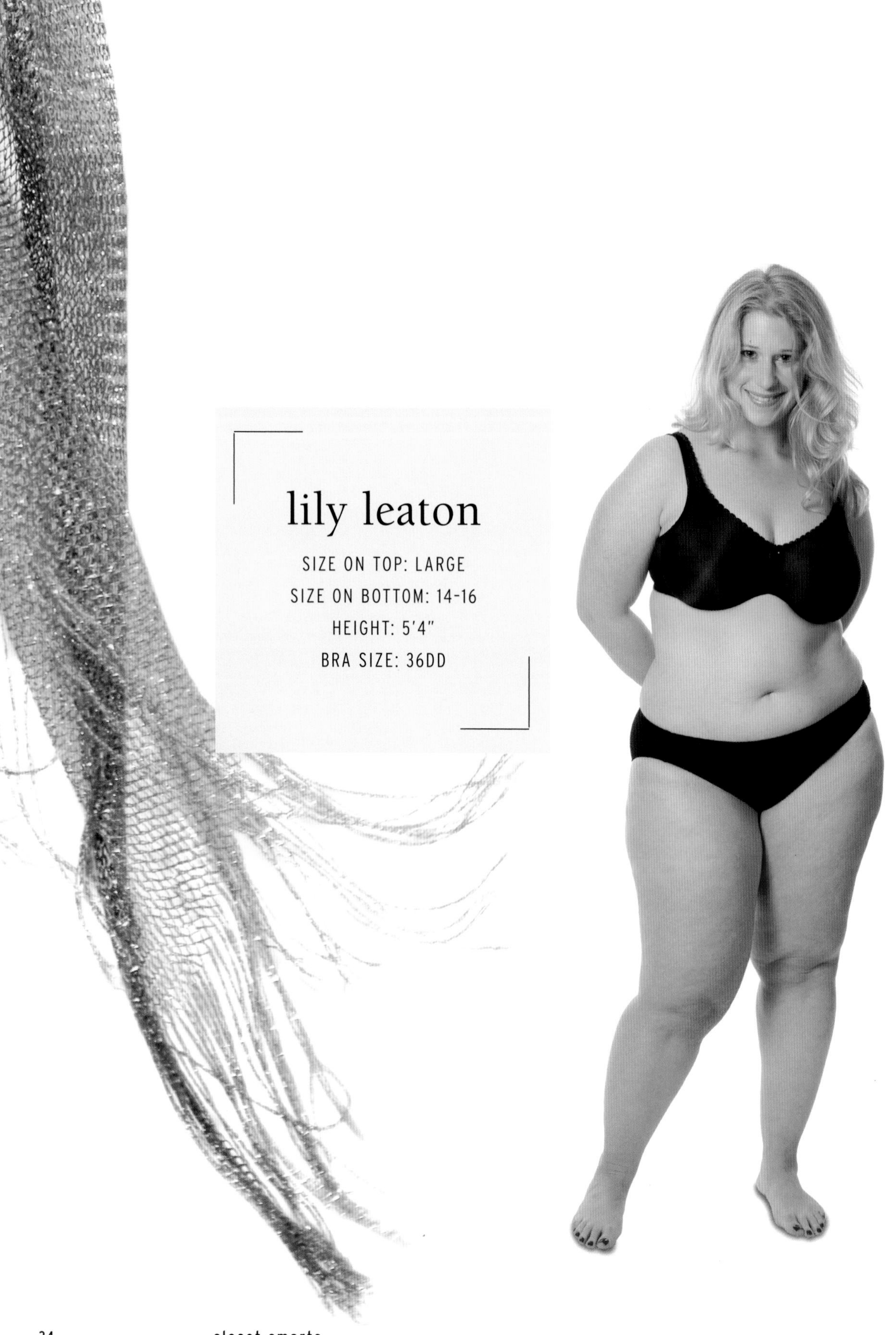

lily leaton

SIZE ON TOP: LARGE

SIZE ON BOTTOM: 14-16

HEIGHT: 5'4"

BRA SIZE: 36DD

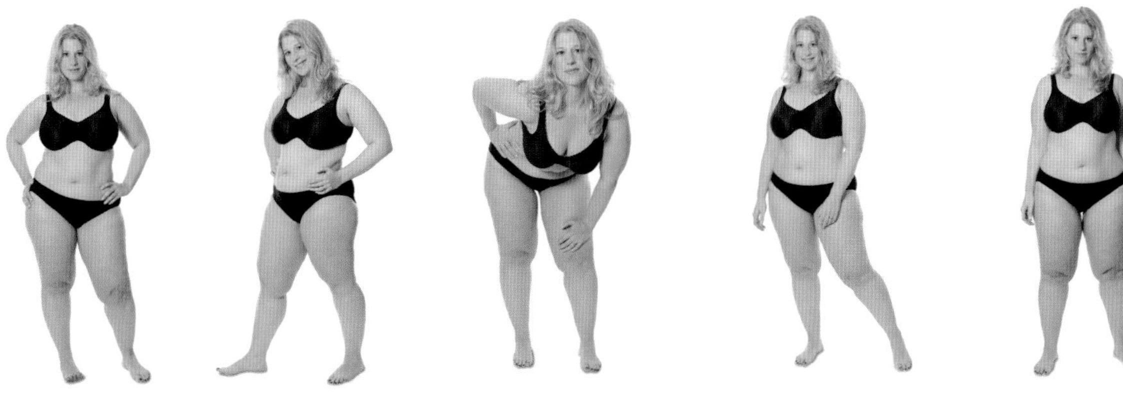

she says:

"When I look in the mirror, my biggest challenge is that I focus on the face up, not my entire body. I've learned to not see that which bothers me. I wear black pants 99.9 percent of the time, and on top, I tend to gravitate toward solids. I always feel most attractive and comfortable in black. I feel I look slimmer in black, and it complements my blonde hair and fair complexion. Black, or dark colors in general, seem to help minimize my large breasts and tush."

i say:

"Lily is the classic plus-size beauty, but she stands to gain from really focusing on more than her pretty face and actively creating a shape for her whole figure, rather than hiding behind monochromatic outfits. There's no fun in that! She can do both—emphasize her lovely face and wear prints and colors and stylish, well-fitting clothes. The trick is in finding pieces that actually hug her body's shape (which has nice curves) in fabrics stiff enough to show off those curves without pulling, rippling, or bulging in the wrong places. She has the additional challenge of being a petite. Finding the right petite styles will go a long way in not overwhelming her shape in too much fabric, which has the double negative effect of making her look bulkier than she truly is and hiding her sexy curves, one of her best assets as far as I'm concerned!"

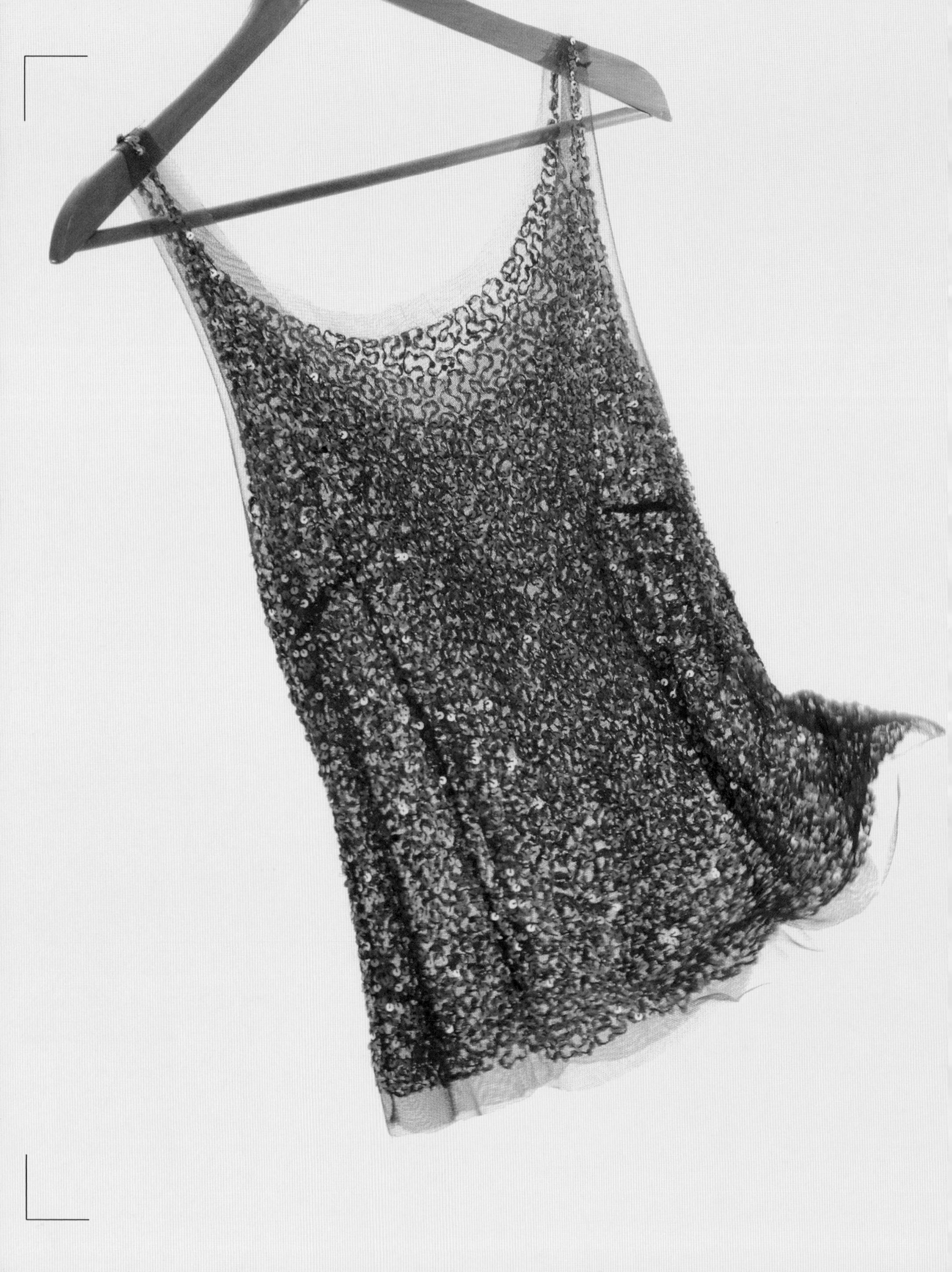

part one: THE UPPER HALF

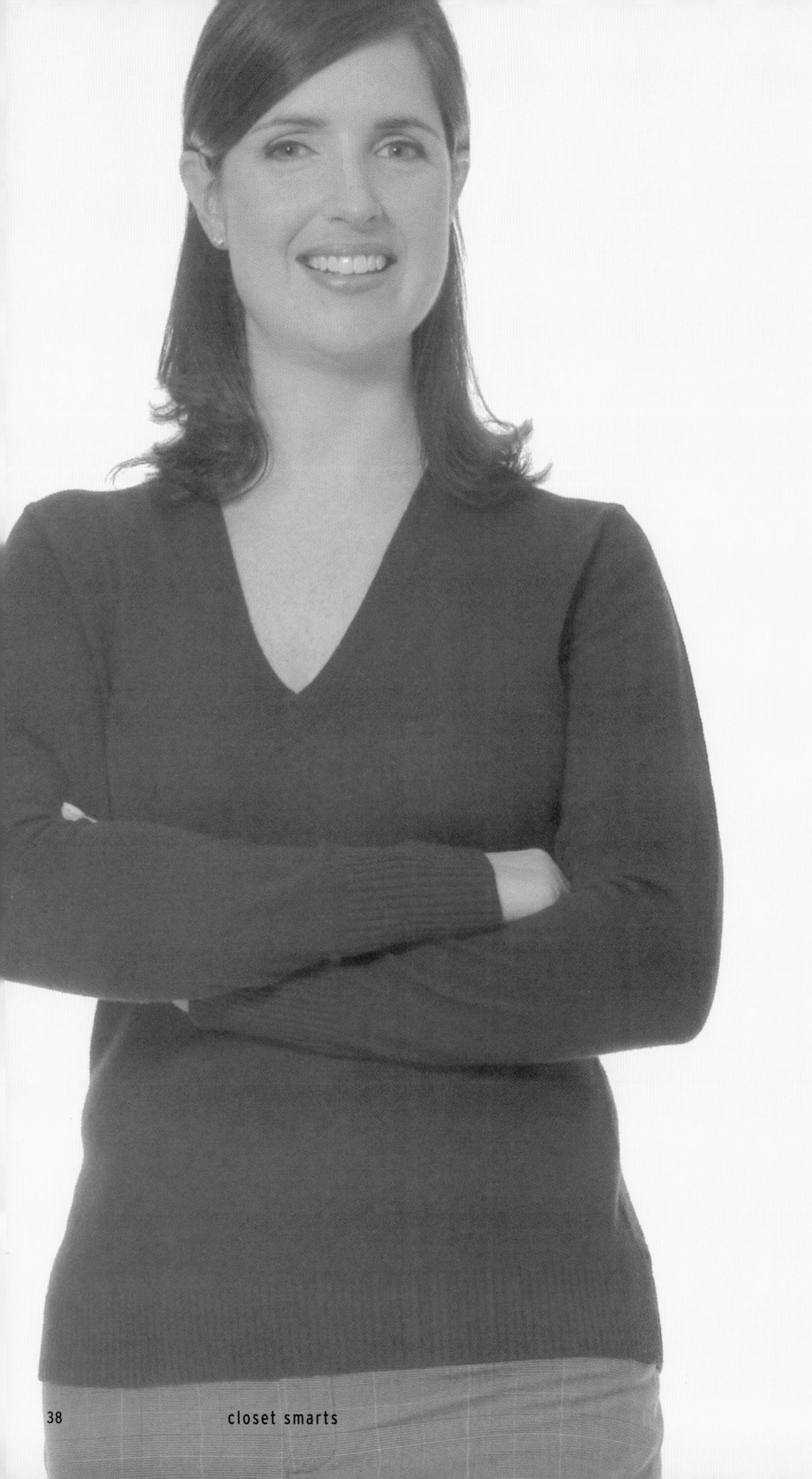

CHAPTER TWO

2

the battle of the neckline

Taking the Plunge

In this chapter, where we start work on the upper half, we begin by addressing an age-old battle about the neckline, captured in a comparison of the turtleneck approach versus the V-neck approach. Whether you've got big boobs or no boobs; whether you are tall, short, or of average height; have a belly, back fat, or love handles to hide; an hourglass waist or no waist, we'll take a look at how you can look your best and show off your best assets while hopefully steering pretty far clear of your attachment to the turtleneck. Don't cry yet. Chin up, and let's make the most of your lovely neck!

A Woman's Neck Is a Thing of Beauty, or The Tragedy of the Turtleneck

I have to say, in all my experience working with women's bodies and women's phobias about their bodies, if there was one universal truth about something that is good for everyone and something that is most likely bad for everyone, it is that V-necks are good, and turtlenecks are bad. And before you fall backward gasping at the thought that your way-too-extensive turtleneck collection is a thing of beauty and how dare I assault it, I ask you to stop and think about that word for a minute—*turtle*neck. Is that really what you want your neck to look like?

Please, everyone, just try not to let your turtlenecks wear you. You deserve to be in charge!

Chances are, you wear turtlenecks because you think they're a great answer to the cold clime you inhabit most of the year. It's a utilitarian thing, right? At least on the surface, that is your philosophy. Lurking just below the surface of that weather rationale is that old instinct that *to cover* is always a better solution than *to expose*. The more you cover up, the less chance of exposing the bad parts! Don't we all feel safer when our clothes hide the real shapes and sizes of our bodies? Along that line of thinking, if the turtleneck is black, all the better! Because if you dress head to toe in black, isn't that slimming?

Listen, I am here to tell you that, like wearing those running shoes with your otherwise smart suit as you commute to work, there are some utilitarian fashion choices that I just cannot call *fashion* choices. They are just *bad* choices. But don't just take my word for it. Instead, let me show you the difference between the fabulous look of the V-neck—the way it opens up your face, draws attention to a universally attractive place on a woman, and creates the basis of a sophisticated and subtly sexy silhouette—and the poor excuse for an article of clothing a turtleneck really is. There are a few people who *can* wear turtlenecks to good effect, but they are few and far between, and they are not most of us.

2

WHO REALLY *CAN'T* WEAR TURTLENECKS?

I think the A number one candidates for *never* wearing turtlenecks are women with larger breasts. Why? Because a turtleneck, besides covering up one of the most attractive and potentially slimming parts of a large-breasted woman's body, her décolletage, creates the unseemly appearance of a uniboob—usually in one giant block of color that does nothing to break up the lines of the upper half. Let's take a look at Lily and Yvette as examples.

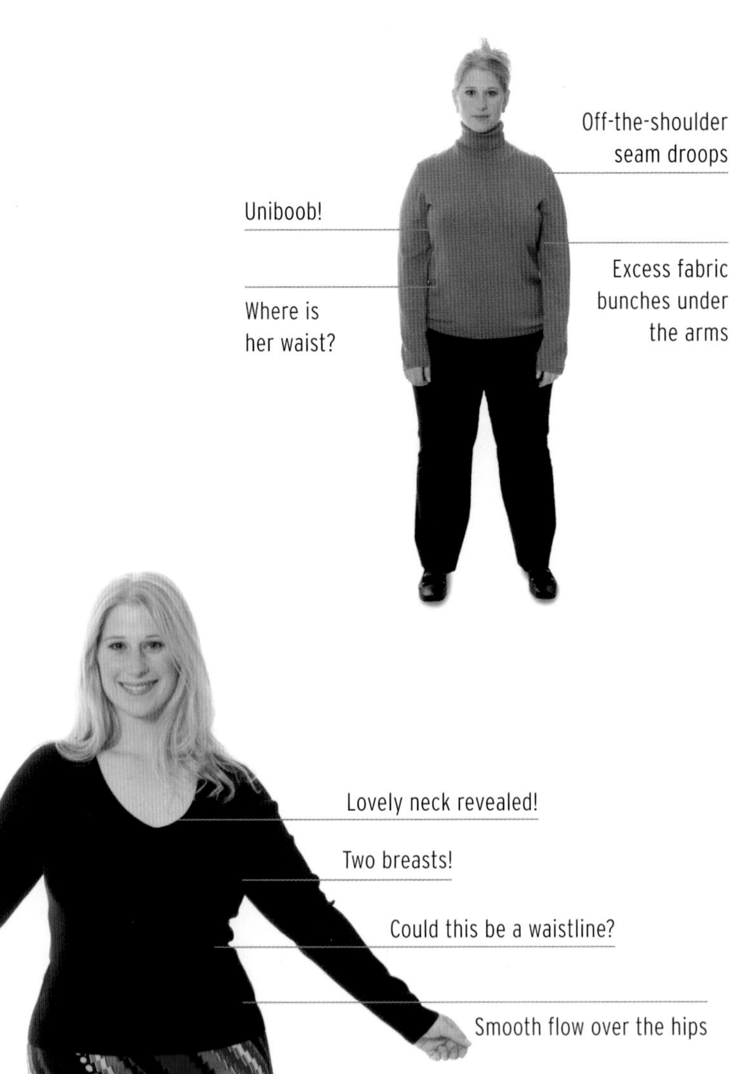

lily before

What's bad about this pretty pink item, you ask? Wrong question, I say. The real question is, what's *good* about it? Is Lily really wearing this, or is it wearing her? Where is she in this giant block of raspberry? Can we see a waist? Curves of any kind? A defined bust? All I see is lots of drapey fabric, that, if anything, drapes in the wrong places and looks droopy. As Lily probably thought when she put it on, "this covers up my problem areas" (unsightly rolls, bulges, a belly). But it does so without *enhancing* any part of Lily either. It's a bad tradeoff–one that is never worth it. That is why I say, the right question to ask of any garment you don is, what is it doing *for* me?

By contrast, let's take a look at the way a V-neck looks on the top of an outfit that Yvette and Lily might wear.

lily now

Here, Lily wears a black V-neck cotton sweater that has a bit of Lycra and is therefore **FITTED THROUGH THE BODICE**, hugging her curves. It is made of a substantial enough fabric that it, combined with the Lycra effect, smoothes over her lumps and bumps. We see the suggestion of her bust's curves, as well as the outline of the narrowest part of her body—the empire waist (just below the bust), and, of course, the **CURVY WAISTLINE** itself. Paired with a **COLORFUL A-LINE SKIRT** that brushes over her hips and a **REFINED HEEL**, Lily is sporting all the coverage she needs in terms of her problem areas, but the look is much more **SOPHISTICATED, SEXY, AND FEMININE**. The overall effect is the appearance of a more shapely top half for Lily. The V-neck draws the eye toward Lily's face and neck and opens up the whole outfit from top to bottom rather than overwhelming her in a swath of color that may well cover over everything, but does so with very little grace or imagination.

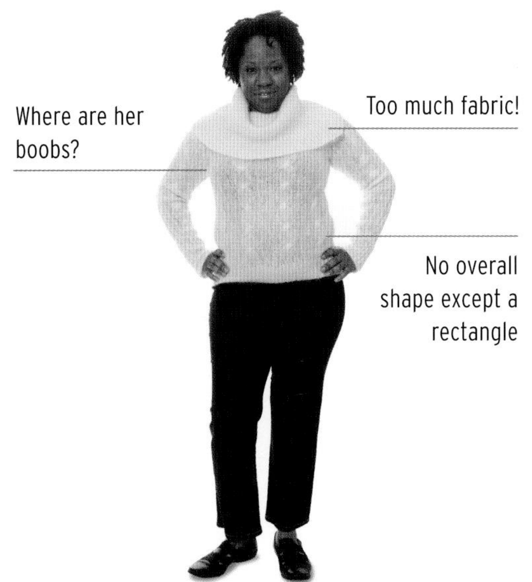

yvette before

Yvette here dons a cowl-necked sweater in the attempt to achieve some reprieve from the otherwise strangling look of the traditional turtleneck. She is sensitive about her neck due to some thyroid swelling and doesn't like to wear things too close to her face as they tend to emphasize her neck's width. But I must ask again, what is this swath of fabric really *doing* for Yvette? What is it that we see? The cream color is nice with her skin, but the whole top of her is just one big block of undefined uni-torso, starting with her boobs and following with the rectangle that this sweater makes of what could be a shapely midsection. True, this type of sweater may cover up a belly, but it's covering everything else as well, and ultimately, it does nothing to *enhance* Yvette's shape, or help create a more attractive shape.

Tasteful cleavage

Narrow waist with empire faux wrap

Belly smoothed over

Flattering cut blends with hips

yvette now

In Yvette's case, the goal is the same. We want to show some of Yvette's **CURVES**—in their smoothest possible light, of course—without simply swathing them in so much material that she ends up looking heavier or thicker than she actually is. The V-neck is a gem for achieving such effect. This faux wrap top works on many levels, but first and foremost, vis-à-vis its V-neck, it **OPENS UP YVETTE'S FACE AND CHEST**. It keeps extra fabric away from her neck (a sensitive area), and shows just the slightest suggestion of **CLEAVAGE** (ever so tastefully). The empire wrap style cinches at the narrowest part of Yvette's torso (just below the bust, again, the empire waist), and skirts out below to **MASK HER BELLY**. Combined with a **CURVE-HUGGING** fluted denim skirt (a fabric heavy enough to smooth out lumps and bumps), which is flared at the knee to **ADD PROPORTION** at the hip, and a refined heel, we see the flip side of what Yvette considers "problem" curves (weight). All we see here are **SEXY AND VOLUPTUOUS CURVES** that are proportioned evenly between Yvette's shoulders, hips, and ankles. Flesh shows in all the right places (chest/face, wrists, calves, and ankles), and Yvette has gone from looking thick-waisted and covered up to looking pretty, sexy, and voluptuous. Which look would you prefer?

WHO *CAN* WEAR TURTLENECKS, BUT WITH CAUTION?

If you're desperate to find a good rationale to wear your collection of turtlenecks, here are a few possibilities. If you happen to be concerned with looking too straight up-and-down (read: not curvy) and perhaps even unbooby, especially if you're on the taller side, a turtleneck with a little Lycra and even some ribbing texture can add or emphasize curves where you haven't much to show for yourself. Let's take a look at our skinny Minnie, Deborah, as an example. As always, even in the best-case scenario, there is a *right* way and a *wrong* way. I don't hedge from my position that turtlenecks are dangerous tools and should be used sparingly and with grave consideration.

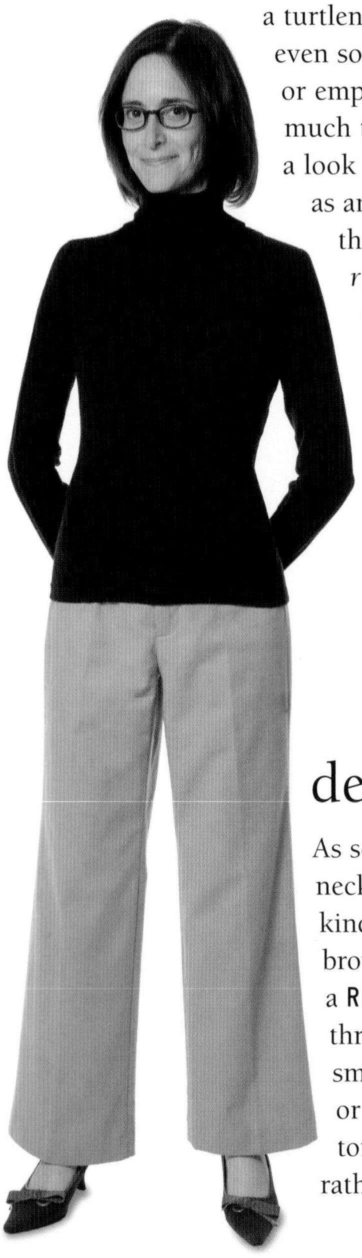

deborah before

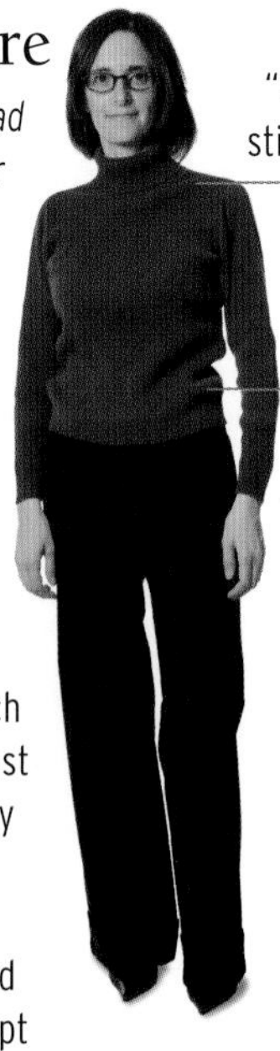

Our first example is the *bad* version of a turtleneck for Deborah. This is your classic ribbed turtleneck, which all of you probably have at least 10 of because they are so cheap and they come in so many different colors! If you are like most people, you got three or four of them for $9.99 each when they went on sale last February, and the February before that, and the February before that. And rather than replace the old with the new, you have kept them *all* because they're warm, right? These cotton-ribbed turtlenecks are absolutely the *worst*. They don't hold their shape, so they quickly bag under the arms and at the sides. They have *way* too much fabric. The wide rib doesn't work on most folks (it just *adds* girth). And the neck is so high, there is no chance any skin will accidentally be revealed around your lovely face. You will truly have a *turtle* neck when you don one of these. As we can see in this picture, bulging fabric does nothing for Deborah's slight frame, even as her goal is to add a little substance to it and avoid looking too skinny. This is *not* the answer. A good turtleneck look for her, however, is possible, as we'll see in the next photo.

"Head on a stick" effect

Too much bunchy fabric

deborah now

As someone on the slightly taller side, Deborah can use a **SLIM-FITTING**, lower-necked, narrow-ribbed turtleneck to cultivate a sophisticated Katharine Hepburn kind of look–the **TALL SLEEK LOOK**, as we see pictured here. This *fitted* mocha brown turtleneck, paired with some beige wool boucle cuffed pants and a **REFINED** brown wool heel, has the overall effect of **SHOWING SOME CURVE** through her bustline (she is a 34B after all), **CINCHING HER WAIST**, and flowing smoothly into a wider-legged pant that avoids making her look too skinny, or overwhelmed by fabric. With Deborah's olive coloring, brown hair, and tortoise eyeglass frames, she makes this turtleneck look like a fashion *choice*, rather than a utilitarian necessity.

WHO ARE THE *BEST* CANDIDATES FOR TURTLENECKS?

If you're tall and slim, turtlenecks won't look as tragic on you as they do on most of us. Sara, as one of our taller models, can choose this option for a sophisticated turtleneck look, and perhaps enters turtleneck territory with less trepidation because she is also for the most part slender (versus skinny or bulky) through the midsection. Her height can help balance out the wads of material a turtleneck imparts to most frames. See the photo on the right to find out how Sara can pull the look off.

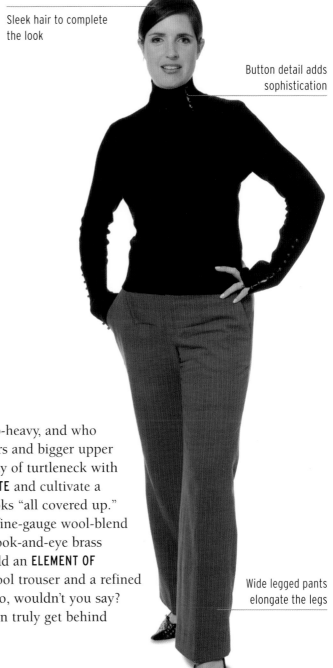

Sleek hair to complete the look

Button detail adds sophistication

Wide legged pants elongate the legs

sara now

As someone who feels she tends to look top-heavy, and who expresses concern about her "wide shoulders and bigger upper body," Sara can use a **SLEEKER-FITTING** variety of turtleneck with wide-legged pants to **EVEN OUT HER SILHOUETTE** and cultivate a **SOPHISTICATED LOOK**, rather than one that looks "all covered up." In the photo to the right, she dons a black fine-gauge wool-blend turtleneck with Lycra—embellished with hook-and-eye brass buttons at the neckline and lower arm to add an **ELEMENT OF INTEREST**—along with a wide-legged grey wool trouser and a refined black heel. She looks absolutely Greta Garbo, wouldn't you say? This is one of the only turtleneck looks I can truly get behind and cheer. Yeah Sara!

Neck brace look

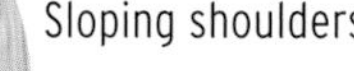

sara before

For comparison's sake, here's Sara in a more overwhelming "warm" turtleneck that I literally had to wrestle out of her wardrobe and forbid her to wear for anything but ski trips. As you can see, though the cream looks delicious with her pale ivory skin and dark hair, the fit makes her look far thicker than she is, turns her bust into a uniboob, and makes her neck look likes she's wearing a brace! Hardly the innocent, *cozy* option she thought it was! And it certainly does nothing to address her concerns about appearing top-heavy.

Square midriff

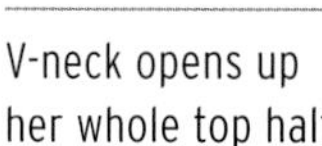

Perfect proportion head to toe

sara now

And to return to where we started, in a comparison of turtlenecks and V-necks, here is the same outfit on Sara minus the bulky turtleneck and opting for the **MORE OPEN LOOK** of a V-neck. This cinnamon-pink cashmere sweater atop her A-line wool skirt and tall leather brown boots **DOES WONDERS** to make Sara's figure appear proportionate at the hip, shoulder, and knee.

2

Morgan, another tall woman in our group, can also help demonstrate a good turtleneck look. But, as is true for everyone when it comes to turtlenecks, she can still make the *wrong* choice as well.

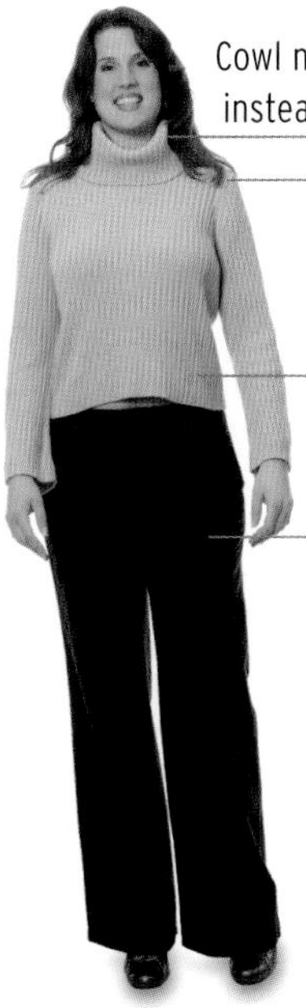

morgan before

This baby blue number, though Morgan adores it and (until I got hold of it) considered it flattering in a "sexy/sloppy kinda way" (she wore it to *work*), is really just more sloppy than anything else. It is too cropped for her height, and that wide-ribbed cotton (which gets too easily stretched out) bags about the arms and body, doing nothing for her midsection—especially when it comes to revealing a waistline. The cowl neck, though it does ease up around her neck, in this case just contributes to the overall look of this sweater as bulky and unkempt.

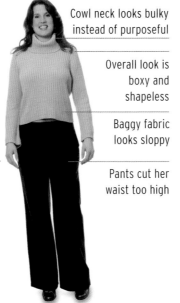

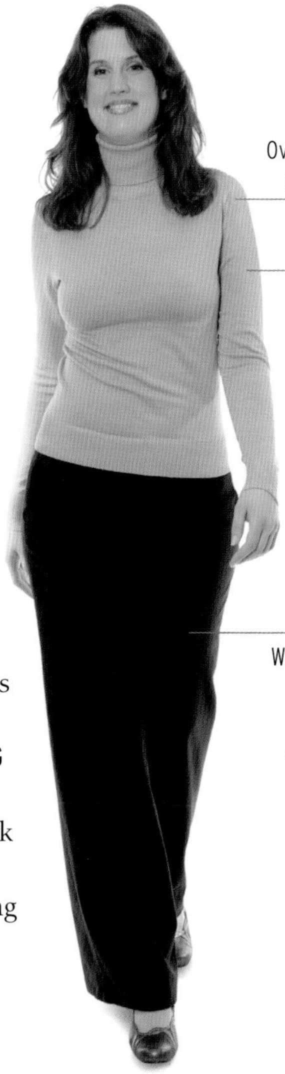

Cowl neck looks bulky instead of purposeful

Overall look is boxy and shapeless

Baggy fabric looks sloppy

Pants cut her waist too high

Overall fit is great

We can see bust and waist

morgan now

Here we see Morgan pictured in a turquoise blue (rather than baby blue), fine-gauge, **FITTED** cashmere turtleneck that **BREATHES SOPHISTICATION**. Coupled with these wide-legged gray wool trousers and a nice heel, Morgan is transformed from her "sexy/sloppy" (read: young) office look into a **REALLY SLEEK AND POLISHED-LOOKING PROFESSIONAL**. The fit, color, and fabric of this sweater all work together here to great overall effect, making this another turtleneck look I can truly get behind and cheer—yeah Morgan! (You see? I *can* be flexible!) My greatest hope is to restrict turtleneck wearing to women whose frames can truly carry the mass of fabric that, for the most part, overwhelms those of typical stature—which is to say, most of us.

Wide-legged pants help to create total proportion of her silhouette

WHAT ABOUT THE REST OF US?

So, let's see, as far as turtlenecks are concerned, we've covered booby, skinny, and tall, but what about the lion's share of us—i.e., those that inhabit that typical place somewhere between a size 8 and 14, and are about 5'2" to 5'4"? Can *we* ever wear turtlenecks? Your best bet, if you've really *got* to wear a turtleneck, is to make it a cowl neck, for much the same reasons I would always recommend a V-neck over most other top options. It keeps the neck open, and (repeat after me) *a woman's neck is a thing of beauty*. (Ask yourself here: Why would you ever *really* have to wear a turtleneck?) Let's look at Amy here as an example.

amy before

This shot shows a more common turtleneck disaster, which truly conjures the image of a turtle. Amy's head literally appears to be perched atop a thick log, adding girth to her face that simply is not there.

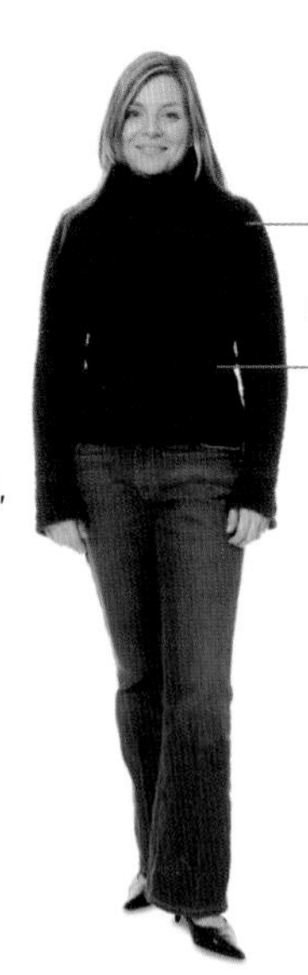

A neck!

Boobs!

Not too much fabric through the waist

A woman's neck is a thing of beauty.

amy now

Here is a great cowl example. We get to see Amy's face and neck, and the sweater also has enough structure to **SHOW HER SHAPE** rather than drape her in material. If you *must* don a turtleneck, go for this look.

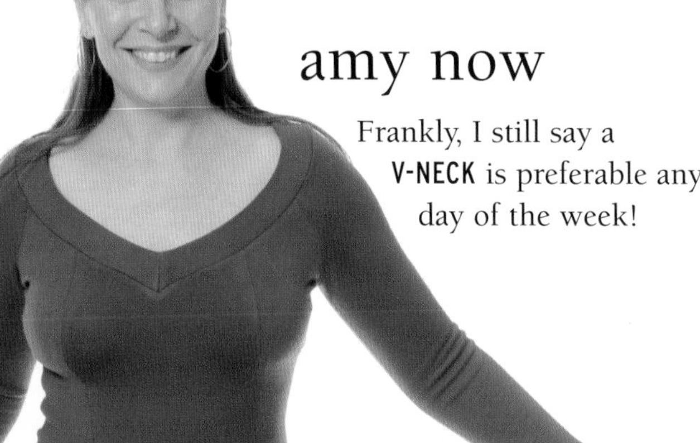

amy now

Frankly, I still say a **V-NECK** is preferable any day of the week!

Need I say or show more? Are you getting it? If you need more evidence about the relative merits of an open-necked top versus the typical appearance of a turtleneck, here is what I have to offer:

sara before
Tragedy

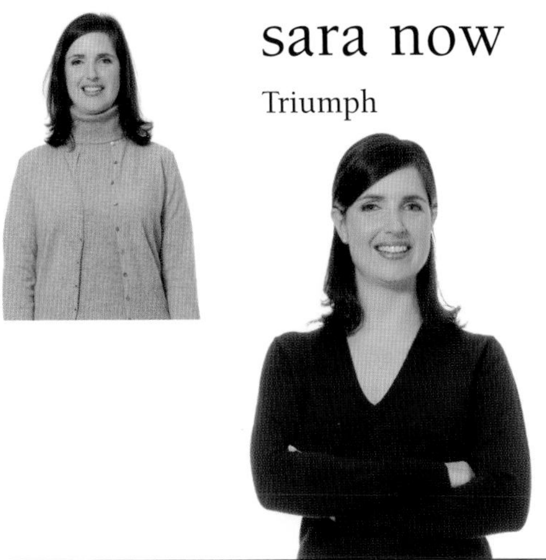

felisha before
Tragedy

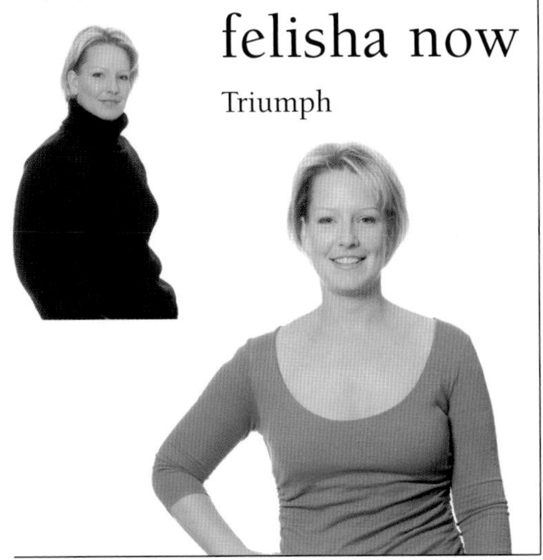

beth before
Tragedy

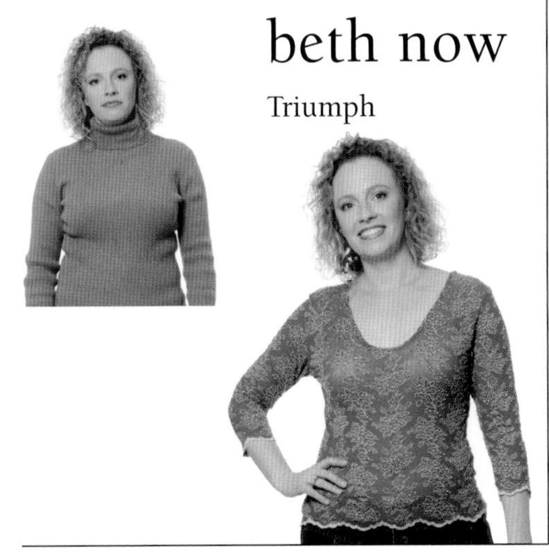

supriya before
Tragedy

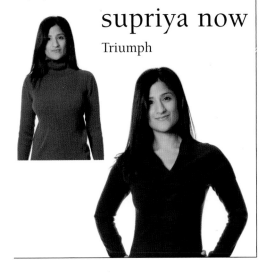

Convinced now?

The Last Word

What should you take away from this chapter? Well, think about your stature: Are you average height? Then for the most part, use turtlenecks with *extreme caution*. Are you chesty? Please, *never* wear one. Skinny? Use them to help you create shape, but be sure not to overwhelm your frame with too much fabric. Buy fitted turtlenecks with darts, seams, ribbing, and Lycra for sure! Are you statuesque? Then have a field day with that old-time movie star glam look, just don't try convincing yourself that a ski sweater is anything you should be wearing to work as a cozy winter alternative. Please, everyone, just try not to let your turtlenecks wear *you*. You deserve to be in charge.

You deserve to be in charge!

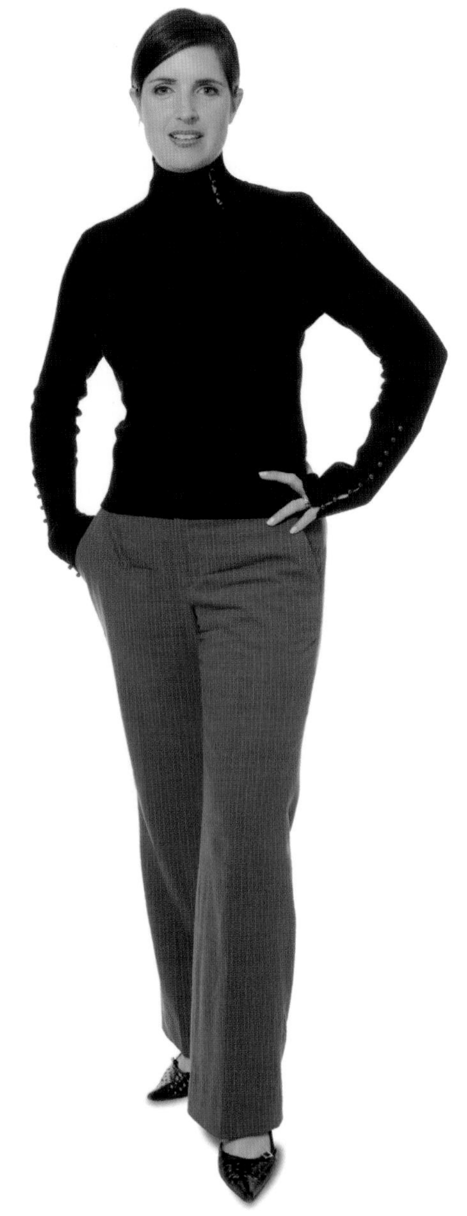

Where to next, then? Why, the neckbone's connected to the . . . shoulder bone! In chapter 3, we will take a closer look at how different shapes of shoulders structure our silhouettes for better and for worse. And of course, there will be plenty of advice about how to achieve your best silhouette.

ULTIMATE NECKLINE STYLE

Here are at-a-glance guidelines to help you make sense of the turtleneck tangle—or escape from it entirely by choosing tops with a more flattering neckline!

1. If you're average height, wear turtlenecks rarely.
2. If you're busty, never wear turtlenecks.
3. If you're skinny, you can wear fitted turtlenecks to help create shape.
4. If you're tall, go for that Hepburnesque black turtleneck look.
5. Whatever your height and shape, a V-neck will be more flattering than a turtleneck any day!

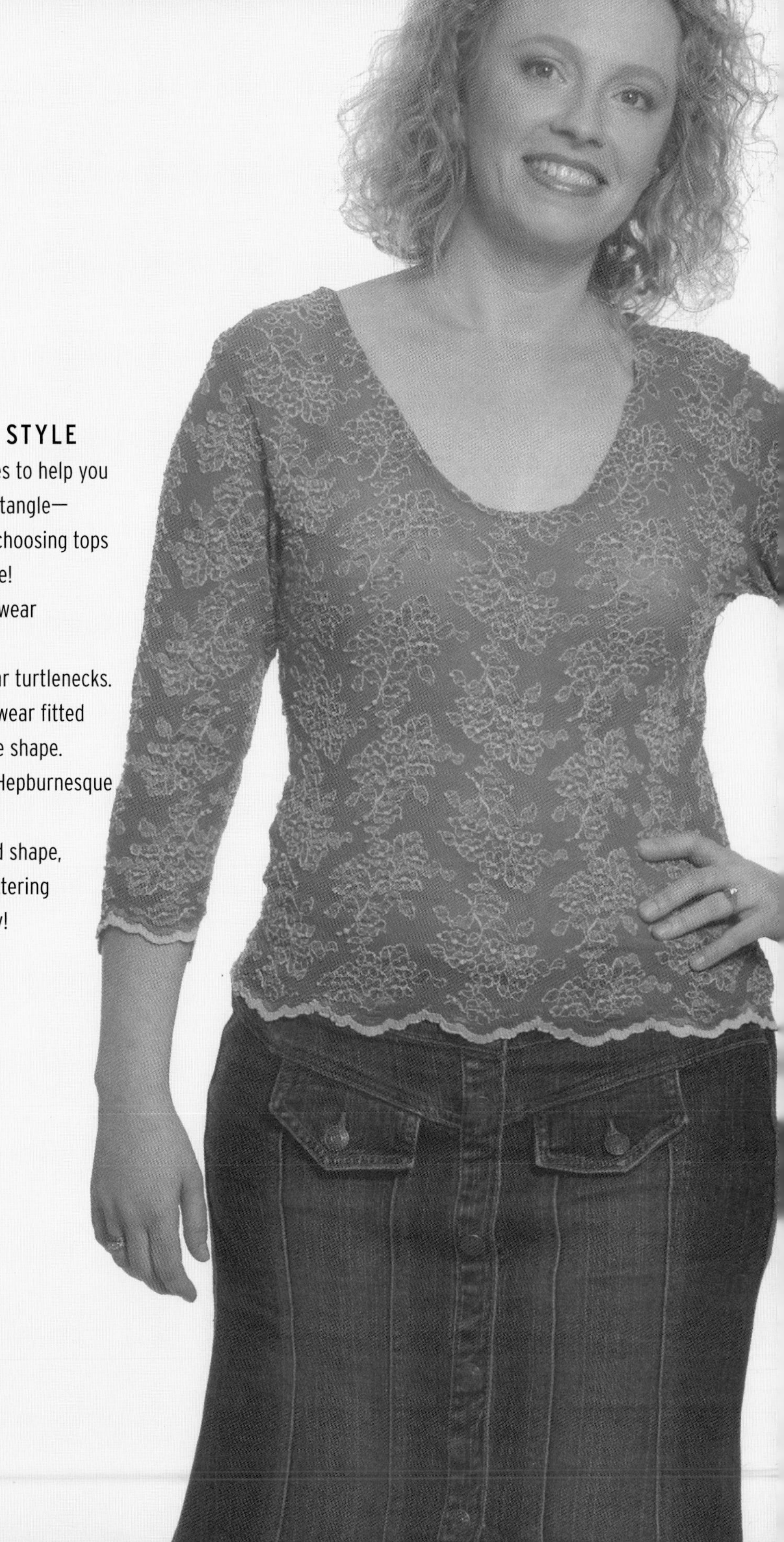

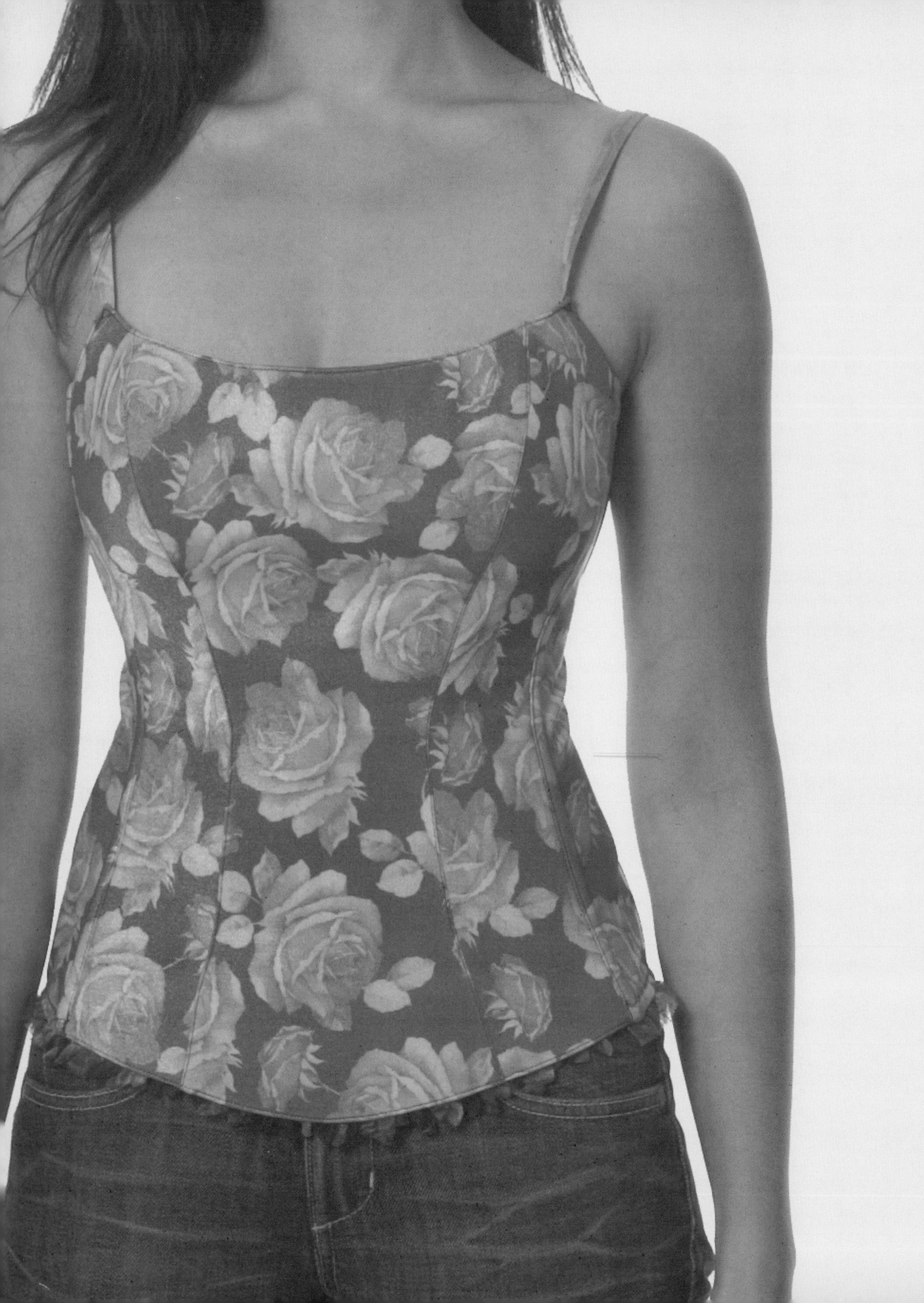

CHAPTER THREE

3

create your own shape

Standing on the Shoulders of Giants

Moving on, we make it as far as the shoulder. Who would think an innocent thing like the top of our arms could have such variety of shapes and such power over the entire structure of our upper halves? I speak as one who has been obsessed with her rounded, sloping, broad, football-player shoulders for years and years. Perhaps this obsession would be better characterized by tears and tears, cried in dressing rooms as I battled to squeeze into petite-sleeved, delicate little blouses and cute little sweaters and jackets, only to have my arms squeezed like salamis in their casings and my upper body immobilized. What I wouldn't give for some tiny little square, skinny arm-toppers... but alas, it was not in the genes. But that doesn't mean I have to settle for looking big-shouldered all the time!

In this chapter, I will show you how to create your own upper-body shape, whether you are broad-shouldered like me or narrow-framed, square or round, heavy or skinny, smooth or muscular. For the most part, in this chapter we will look at the power of the jacket to add structure to our upper halves, in the proportion our silhouettes want and need. In the next few chapters, we will look at other strategies for revising our tops and editing our silhouettes into shapes we can live with.

The Shoulder Crisis: Rounded and Sloped

Why is it a crisis? Perhaps because it is my own figure pet peeve, but also because the shoulder rarely gets the attention it deserves—a mistake, since it can ruin an otherwise perfectly nice silhouette. The shape of a shoulder can really affect the overall look of an outfit on our frames, and if we don't pay attention to it, we will pay in one way or another.

To begin with the more difficult masquerade, if you are a sloping- or round-shouldered gal, there are many things to look out for and many strategies for creating a bit more structure to your top half. Coming off our V-neck rant in chapter 2, the easiest, quickest fix is to do your best to avoid crewnecks. These are the kind of round, high-necked tops most stereotypically found on the standard T-shirt. The appearance of a rounded silhouette is exaggerated—not what you need!—by more round lines, which are what crewnecks and higher scoopnecks foster.

Next on the list of to-dos (or don't dos, as the case may be), of course: Choose *V-necks* instead of scoops or crews! Third trick? Watch out for the shoulder seam on all your tops; danger awaits those who let this detail slide. Keep those seams where they were meant to be, *on* your shoulder, not off the side of your shoulder. (No raglan sleeves!) Fourth? Add a structured jacket as your top layer. The jacket device is one of the most reliable and easy ways to insure that you have control over your silhouette. Don't miss out on this simple fashion option!

So to showcase good and bad options for sloping and rounded shoulders, let's look to Felisha, Lily, and Yvette as examples. Felisha is more of a sloping-shouldered gal, while Lily and Yvette both have a bit more of the solid rounded thing going on.

felisha before

Here is Felisha in a drawstring tunic top—exactly the wrong look for someone concerned with adding a bit more perpendicular shaping to her sloping shoulders. This top has no shoulder seam at all, and combined with the soft scoop neck, made even softer by the drawstring detail, we end up *enhancing* Felisha's sloping/ rounded look rather than ameliorating it. Though this effect may work very well to soften up someone with an overly bony top half (we'll get to that later), it has left Felisha with too much softness where she needs just the opposite. So how do we fix it? What are her options? There are a few, as we mentioned earlier. The easiest one is to switch out the scoop neck for the V-neck, and apply a highly structured jacket, as we do in the "after" photo. Presto change-o, take a look at her now!

Scoop neck emphasizes roundness

Absence of seam enhances the slope effect

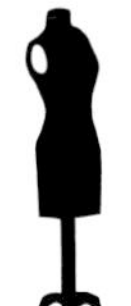

closet smarts: SLOPING SHOULDERS

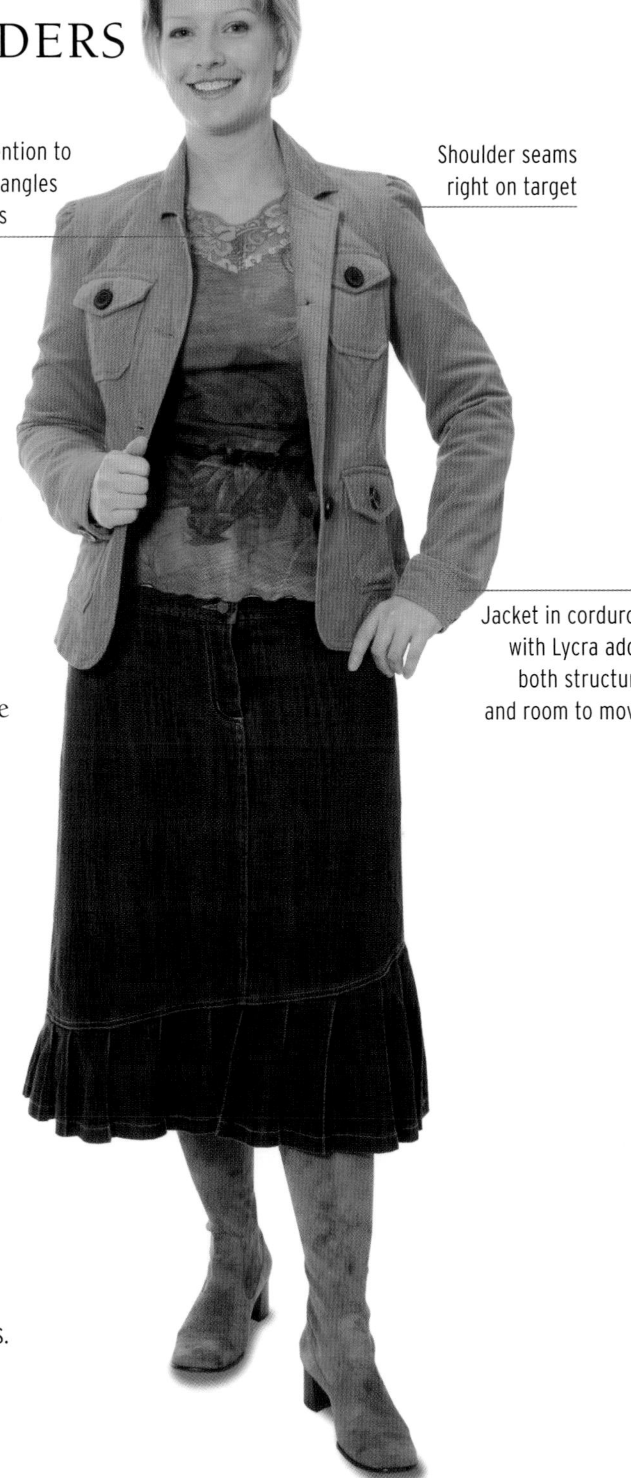
V-neck draws attention to neck and creates angles rather than circles
Shoulder seams right on target
Jacket in corduroy with Lycra adds both structure and room to move

felisha now

What a difference a jacket can make to correct a sloping shoulder! Here, thanks to a jacket with **STRUCTURED SHOULDERS** and subtle padding, Felisha looks as top **PROPORTIONATE** as the most genetically blessed amongst us. Same girl, seemingly different shape. It can be that easy. But, as with most fashion options, it can also go wrong. We've got to keep in mind all the tricks of the trade simultaneously, so that we pick the *right jacket*, the *right shoulder* seam, the *right neckline*, and blend them all to **BEST EFFECT**.

SMART TIPS FOR ROUND SHOULDERS

If you have sloping or rounded shoulders, you'll give your top half more structure if you use these tips.

1. Avoid crewnecks and high scoopnecks.
2. Choose V-necks instead of scoops or crews.
3. Keep shoulder seams on your shoulders.
4. Add a structured jacket as your top layer.

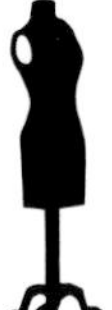

closet smarts:
ROUNDED SHOULDERS

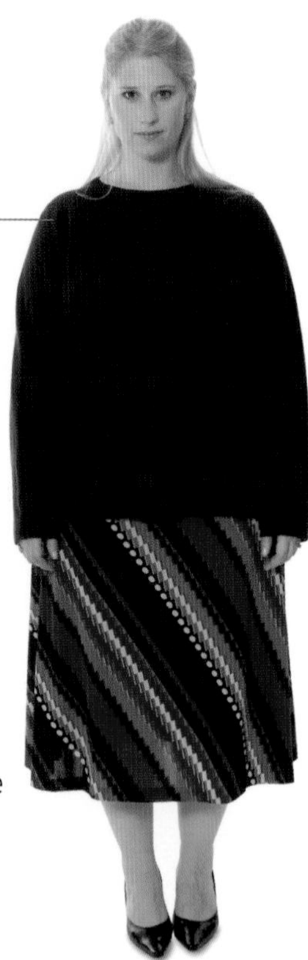

Shoulder seams are on her arms!

lily before

Here is Lily in her crew-necked, not to mention *shapeless* shirt, which does absolutely nothing for her rounded shoulders (but emphasize them, that is). I think she may have thought that this shirt gave her good coverage. (I can't imagine why else it would be in her wardrobe!)

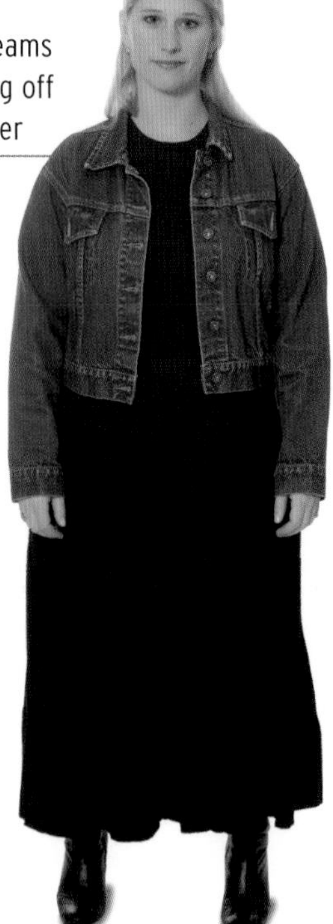

Problem seams are hanging off her shoulder

Choosing the *right* jacket to layer with is as important as the initial instinct to add structure through layering. In this next example, Lily adds a jean jacket, which simply mimics the same rounded shape of her crewneck top; they both have poorly placed shoulder seams.

lily now

Here is a much **BETTER** look for Lily: It pairs the crisp pointed collar of a stretch oxford shirt with a cropped, fitted boxy jacket. (Large-breasted women like Lily can actually use boxy jackets to better effect than most, because their **BUILT-IN CURVES** thwart the usual result, which is to make the wearer look as boxy as her jacket.) This look not only crisps up Lily's top half, adding **GOOD STRUCTURE** to her silhouette, but in keeping her neck and face opened up and framed by soft lilac, it beautifully mixes **SOFTER FEMININE ELEMENTS** with that darker suity look.

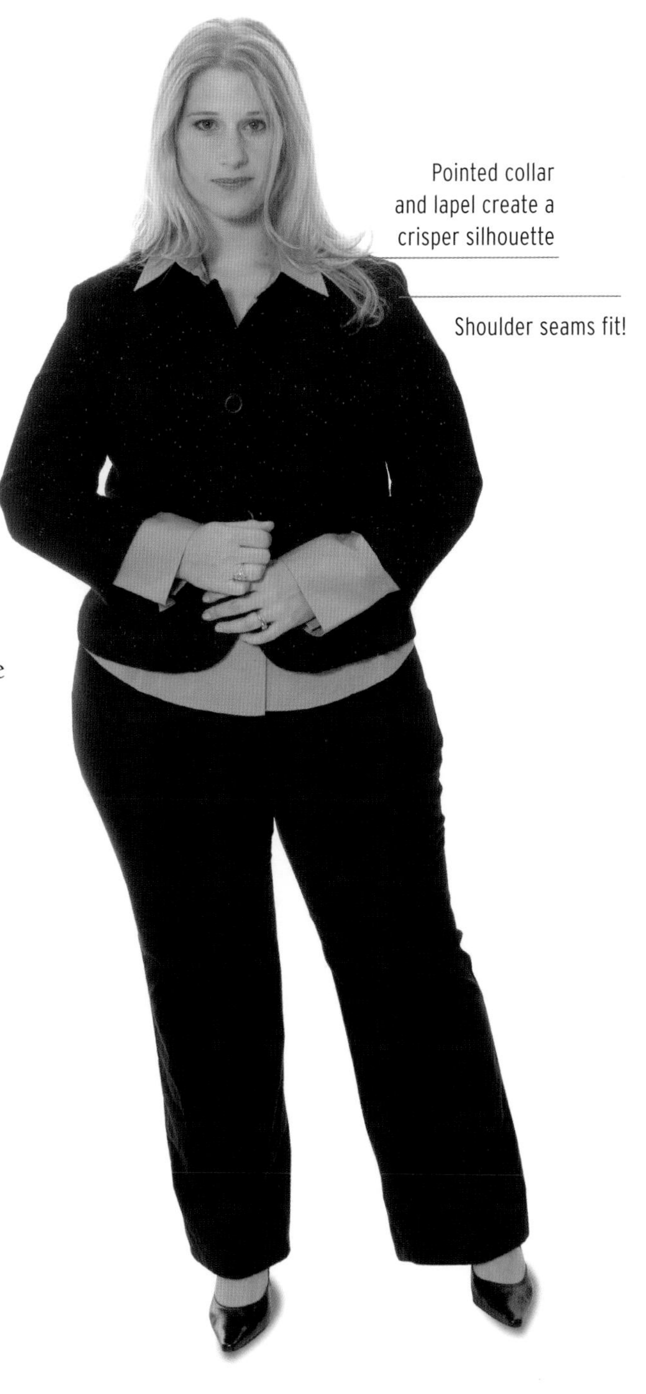

Pointed collar and lapel create a crisper silhouette

Shoulder seams fit!

CLOSET SMARTS STYLE

As I warned on page 54, be aware when trying on any kind of top—and particularly if you have more rounded shoulders—that the seam of your top should fall squarely at the top edge or even a bit inward from your shoulder. Wearing anything that falls off the edge of your shoulder is a sure way to enhance the look of softness and roundness. By contrast, wearing any kind of top that fits your shoulder squarely will help create a more structured silhouette.

closet smarts:
ROUNDED SHOULDERS

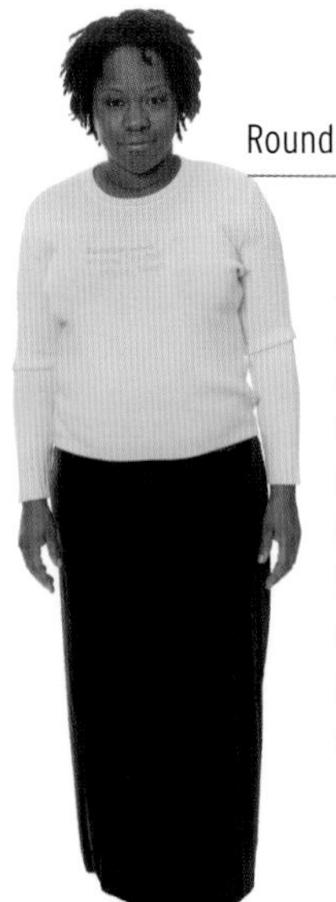

Round=round

yvette before

And what about Yvette, who also struggles with sharpening up her more rounded edges, which are easily accentuated through inattention to shoulder styling? I tell you, the same formula works every time, and that's what's going to make it easy for you once you put this book down. Here is Yvette in an unflattering (read strangling, rounded, and otherwise shapeless) crewneck top.

V-neck also counteracts the round elements of her top half

Structured jacket adds angled proportion to top half

yvette now

Swap out that crewneck for a V-neck, add a **STRUCTURED JACKET** with a fitted shoulder seam, and whala! Yvette's face and chest are opened up as the **FOCAL** points of the ensemble, her larger chest is masked by the shape and drape of the jacket, and her newly squared (and **PROPORTIONATE**) shoulders carry her top half masterfully. The shape of the shoulder in this jacket is what we see as the **DEFINING ASPECT** of Yvette's silhouette, and it balances out the rest of her curves to achieve the proportionate effect we were looking for.

The Other Side of the Shoulder Crisis: Square and/or Bony

From my perspective, this would never be a crisis, but an opportunity to thank my lucky stars on a daily basis! But I must admit that for some, having bony and squarish shoulders is *un*desirable. They feel that their boniness is unfeminine (where feminine is seen as more fleshy and soft-looking), that their square silhouettes are boyish and lacking in curves, or simply that boniness is an unseemly quality for body parts as prominent and important as shoulders are in defining one's shape. So, for those reasons, I must address this problem and sigh deeply, wishing it were mine.

Here we will follow the travails of Sara, who feels that her shoulders are too square and dominating, as well as Deborah and Supriya, both of whom "suffer" from having bonier shoulders.

As we saw in photos back in chapter 2, Sara is a big fan of the twinset (usually with a turtleneck), because she feels there is enough fabric there to soften and round out her top half. She is certainly right about there being enough fabric there to do *something*, though I'm not sure it's "softening" her look in the way she intends it to! A better word might be "padding," but I digress.

Soften square shoulders, don't pad them.

SMART TIPS FOR SQUARE SHOULDERS

If you have square or bony shoulders, give your top half a softer look by trying these tips.

1. Choose soft sweater jackets in darker colors.
2. Choose scoops or crews instead of V-necks.
3. Avoid shoulder seams that fall on your shoulders; go for raglan and other unconstructed sleeves.
4. Experiment with fuller sleeves, like princess sleeves, for a more feminine look.

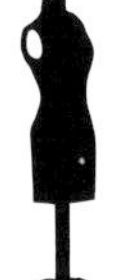

closet smarts: SQUARE SHOULDERS

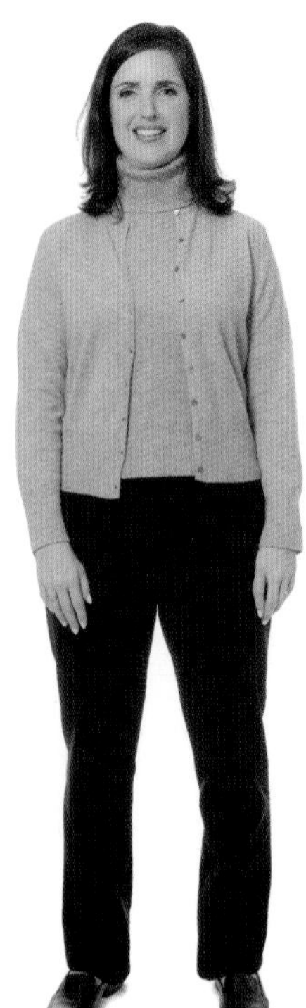

sara before

As I noted in the turtleneck section in chapter 2, this look is totally and completely unflattering to Sara, square shoulders or no. This sweater set is *not* the answer! But what is? For her, I have at least three suggestions. Quite contrary to my advice in the previous section about shoulder seams, those with concerns about squarish shoulders can in fact carry off a top without shoulder seams, more familiarly known as the raglan sleeve (where the sleeve, instead of ending at the shoulder, extends to the collar, attached with slanting seams running from under the arm to the neck).

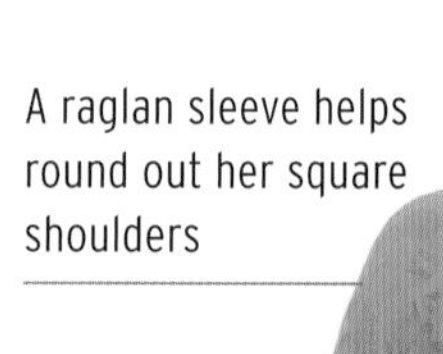

A raglan sleeve helps round out her square shoulders

Fitted through the bust and waistline we see Sara's curves all over!

sara now

Here we see Sara in a zip-front jackety top with a raglan sleeve. It is **NICELY FITTED** throughout the bodice to **ENHANCE HER CURVES** elsewhere, and the raglan cut does quite a good job of softening the squareness of her shoulder while keeping her body proportionate from shoulder to waist.

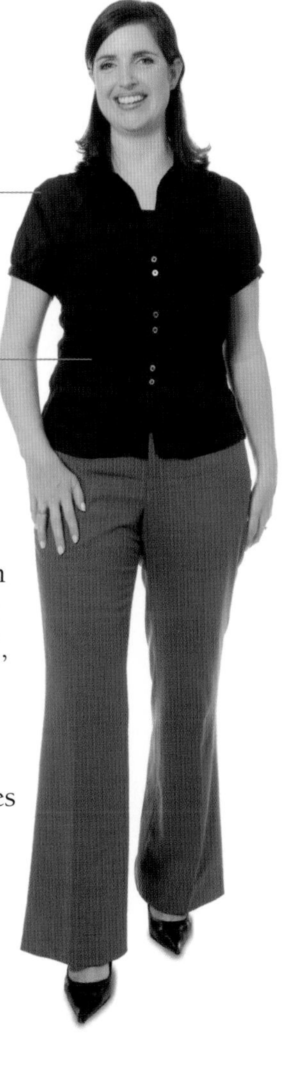
The poofy sleeve
gives roundness
to her shoulders
The darts in the
shirt add shape
to her midsection

sara now

Another option for Sara is to choose a **FEMININE BLOUSY LOOK** with a princess sleeve (i.e., a poof at the shoulder). This look is always **SOFT**, always feminine, sometimes a bit too babydoll, but worn with these shapely wide-legged wool slacks and **REFINED** black heels as Sara does here, she definitely takes it more to the **ELEGANT** side. The blouse is **FITTED** with darts and feminine **CURVES** throughout, which add to the effect she is trying to achieve in softening the appearance of her shoulders.

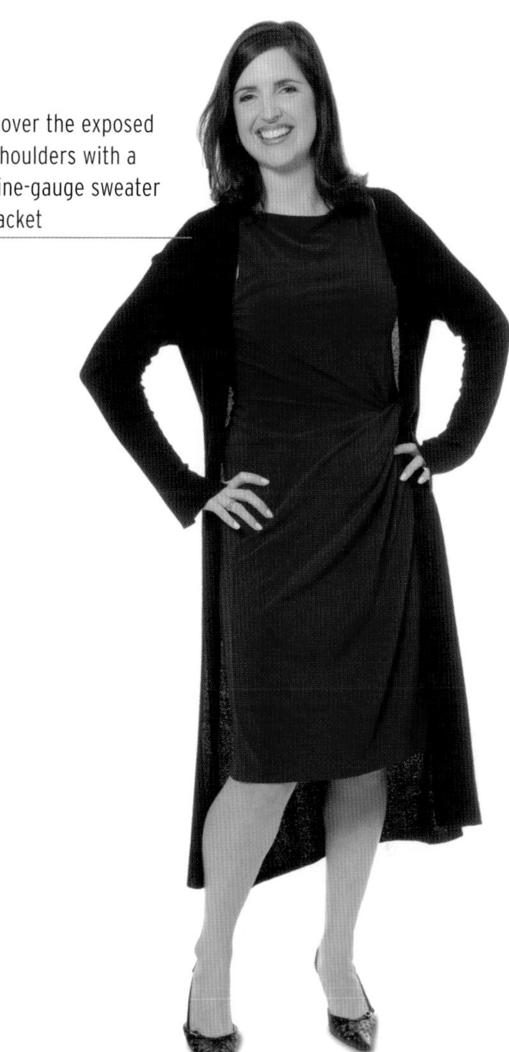
Cover the exposed
shoulders with a
fine-gauge sweater
jacket

sara now

Finally, when Sara dons a **FAVORITE** faux-wrap sleeveless dress, she can avoid fears of appearing too domineering on the top half by **SOFTENING THE LOOK** with this light-gauge sweater jacket. By draping her bare shoulders in a darker fabric, she is able to mask any appearance of their square shape and soften their presence in her overall look.

closet smarts:
SKINNY SHOULDERS

DISGUISING SKINNY SHOULDERS

And what about the bony gals? The best advice I can give right off the bat: Always wear clothes that truly fit the size of your arms and shoulders rather than going larger as an answer to masking thinness. It's hard to hide the fact that you are swimming in fabric, and frankly, I've never seen it look good on anyone, heavy or thin. My advice is the same on both sides of the fence.

What you need to do first and foremost is invest the time in finding tops that really do fit your small size. It's generally true that once you've found a top that fits you really well, you'll find that the brand tends to make similar tops year after year, so always note which brands work on you and make an effort to find them. This can take work, and it is what I do for a living when I shop with people, but once you find your brands, you will have a much easier time of it. Stick with them and rely on them! It's what learning to shop smart is all about, and you'll be less likely to make mistakes in your efforts to mask undesirable features (in this case, boniness). As an example, take a look at Supriya in the following photos.

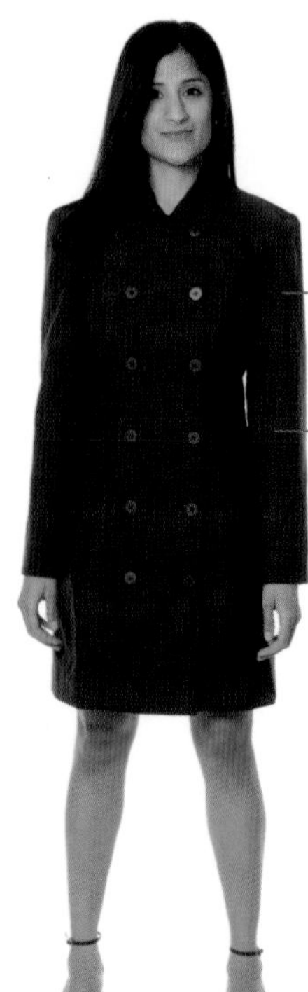

These shoulders are way too large!

We see no shape with this boxy dress

supriya before
Too big!

The peplum waist band shortens her waist a bit, while creating nice shape

The thicker corduroy adds shape without overwhelming

supriya now
This miniaturized jacket really fits!

It's hard to hide the fact that you are swimming in fabric.

Second, unlike many other fashion advisors who seem to suggest the all-or-nothing approach (if you have heavier arms, *never* wear short sleeves, or if you have bony shoulders, *always* cover them), I am more of the mind that where your clothing lies on or cuts across a problem area can make *all* the difference as to how those spots end up looking. This is the approach I have cut my fashion teeth on—that you can actually do a great deal to create the shape of your body with clothing and the right cut and fit. Doubt me? Take a look at these two shoulder-baring tops on Supriya.

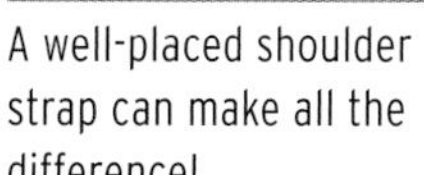

Shoulder shape is really emphasized here

supriya before

Here in the halter top, Supriya's shoulders are emphasized as the line of the halter cuts diagonally across her shoulder inward, exposing the largest possible uninterrupted surface area. Because of this, we get a real look at Supriya's shoulders as is in this shape of top.

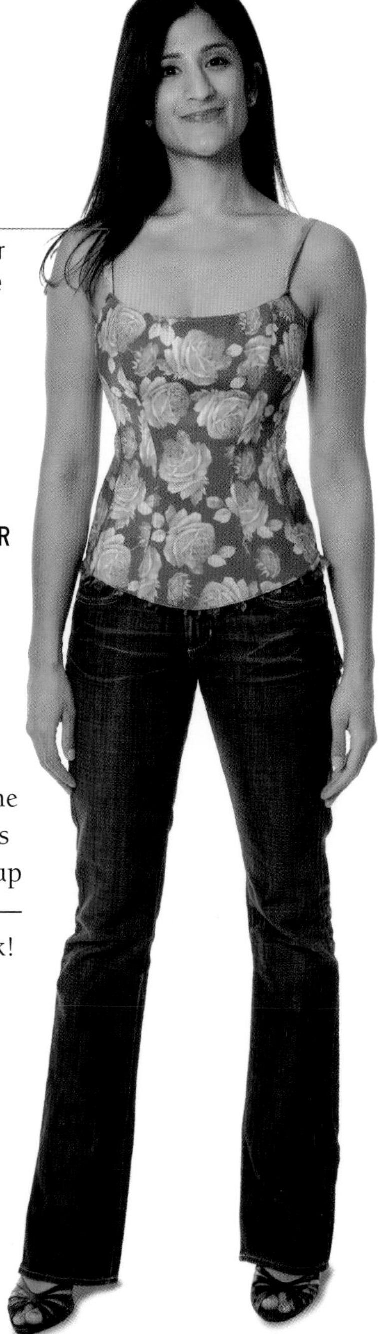

A well-placed shoulder strap can make all the difference!

supriya now

When we look at the **BUSTIER TOP** with a strap that cuts diagonally outward across her shoulder, what we end up seeing is the broken line of that shoulder, the effect of which is to **DISTRACT THE EYE** from the real shape of the shoulder. The focus becomes her chest, which is opened up by the framing of the straps—a **MUCH MORE ATTRACTIVE** look! In both cases, Supriya gets to wear her shoulders bare, but we get a very different impression of their shape.

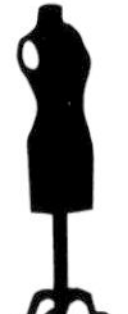

closet smarts:
SKINNY SHOULDERS

For Deborah, who is even tinier than Supriya, her best bet in choosing a sleeveless top is to stick to a thicker strap so as to break up the bony or knobby appearance of her shoulders. Take a look at both of these tops on her.

A thicker shoulder strap creates the illusion of softer, fuller shoulder shape

Spaghetti straps emphasize bony shoulders

deborah before

In this first camisole top, the straps are so thin that they really accentuate her tininess. Her arms look almost stick-like.

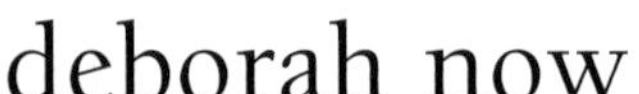

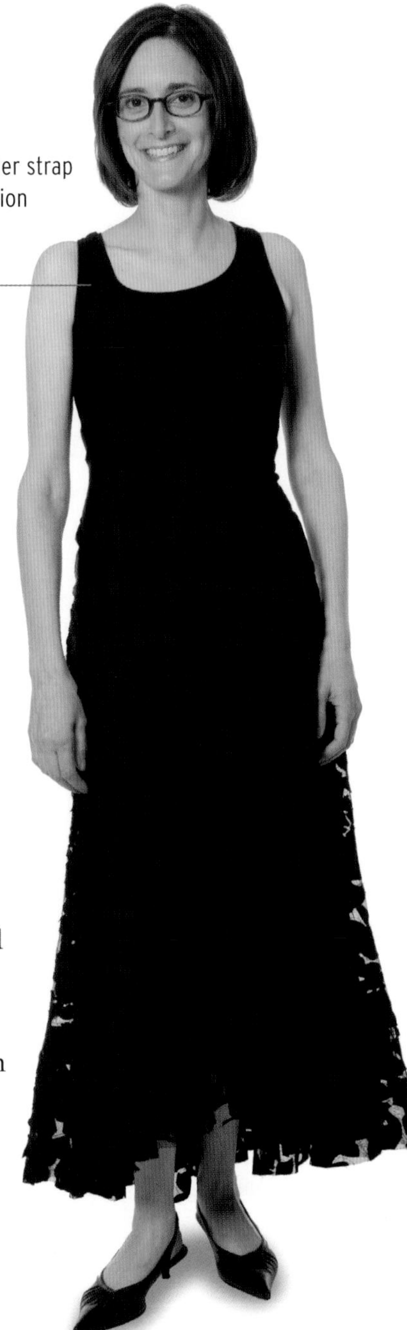

deborah now

This second option really fills out Deborah's top half, and by **HUGGING** the curve of her bust and waist with a **LITTLE LYCRA**, it focuses attention on **CURVES** rather than angles.

As for the opposite instinct, to add fabric to deal with the problem, here are some examples of good- versus ill-fitting jackets in the shoulder department. Deborah is definitely going to do best with a miniaturized jacket (one that is designed to be more decorative and petite than traditionally suity).

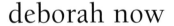

deborah before

Here is the *wrong* look. This jacket is overwhelming on Deborah's frame, though she thought it had an elegant and classic appeal. There are many things I could say about it, and I will later, but for now, notice that the shoulder pad really does not actually work here to pad Deborah's shoulder in the way she desires (to mask her boniness). It just serves to make the jacket look too big on her—almost David Byrnian!

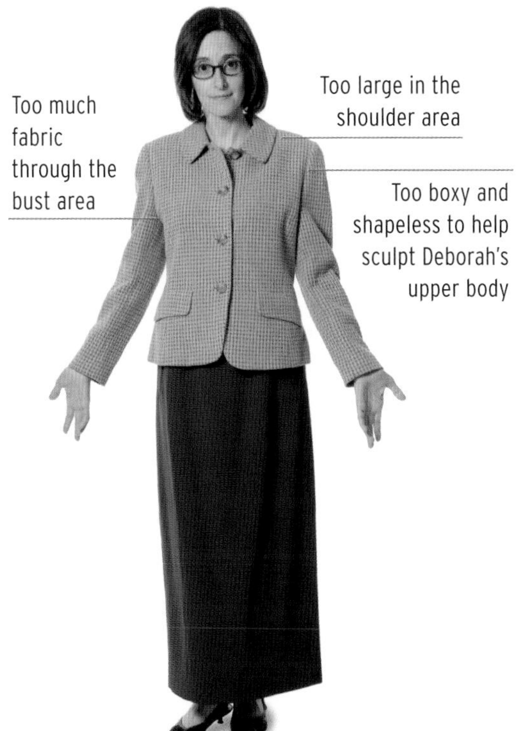

Too much fabric through the bust area

Too large in the shoulder area

Too boxy and shapeless to help sculpt Deborah's upper body

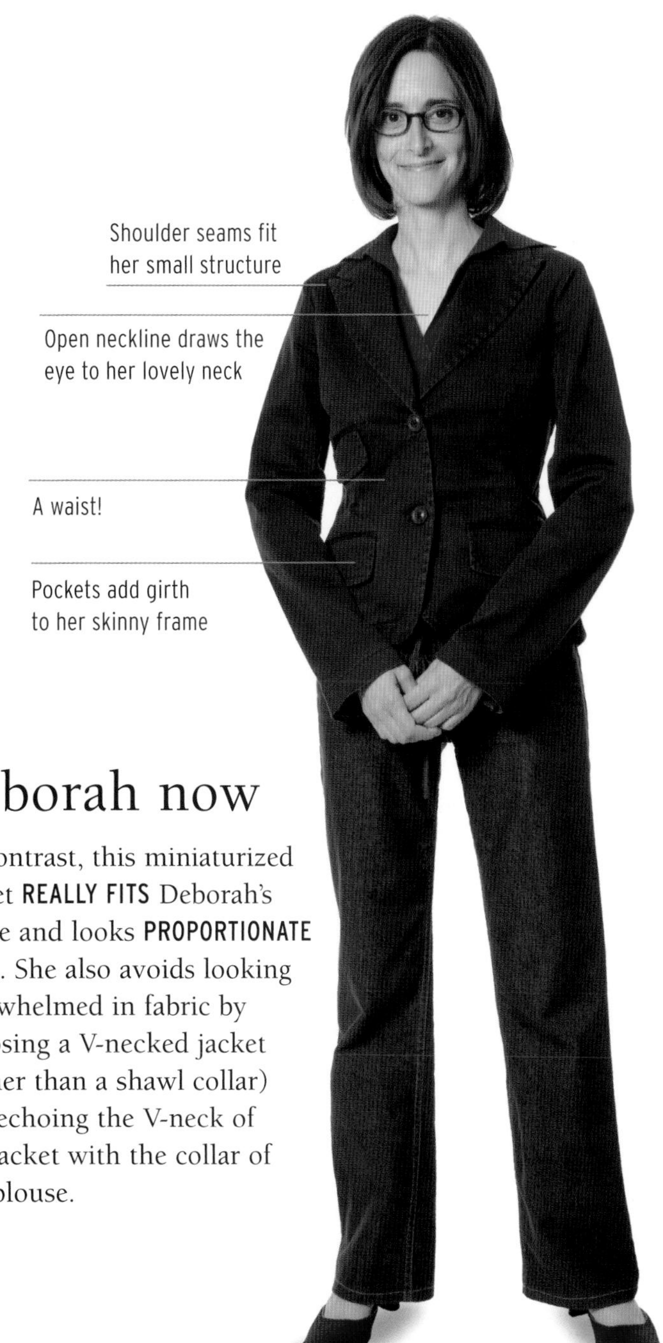

Shoulder seams fit her small structure

Open neckline draws the eye to her lovely neck

A waist!

Pockets add girth to her skinny frame

deborah now

By contrast, this miniaturized jacket **REALLY FITS** Deborah's frame and looks **PROPORTIONATE** on it. She also avoids looking overwhelmed in fabric by choosing a V-necked jacket (rather than a shawl collar) and echoing the V-neck of the jacket with the collar of her blouse.

The Last Word

So, there you have it, strategies for the best and worst shoulder shapes. (I'll let you be the judge of your favorite shape, as I can *not* be objective about this issue!) What's the most important thing to remember? The right answer is *never* simply to swathe anything in fabric to fix it. It just doesn't work for anyone, broad- or narrow-shouldered. Assess your issues and work with the seams and straps of your top pieces. If you are rounded, look for square, if you are square, look for curves. In both cases, *always* look for a proportionate fit, because if your proportions are off, nothing can help you.

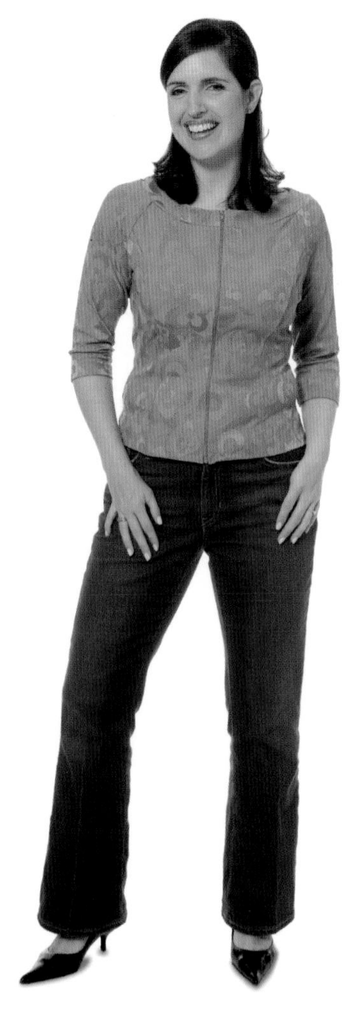

If you are rounded, look for square. If you are square, look for curves.

So what's next? In the next chapter, we'll talk about arms (heavy, skinny, muscular) and how to dress so they look great, whether you're wearing sleeves or—gasp!—daring to bare them. Trust me on this: Try it, you'll like it, no matter what shape your arms are in. Don't believe me? You will after you read chapter 4, and that's a promise!

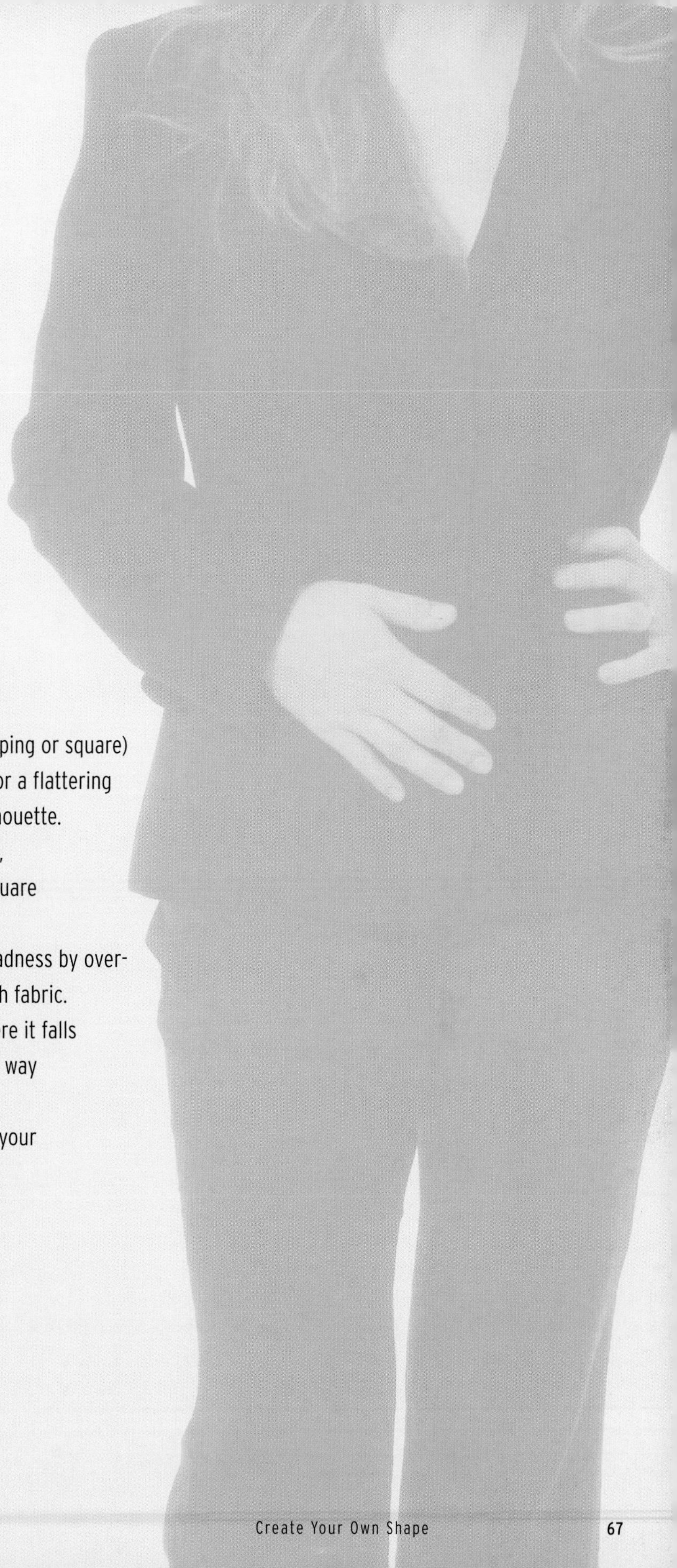

ULTIMATE SHOULDER STYLE

Whether your shoulders are broad (either sloping or square) or narrow (bony or angular), use these tips for a flattering fit and a great-looking, well-proportioned silhouette.

1. If your shoulders are rounded or sloping, look for more structure; if they're too square or bony, look for softer curves.
2. Never try to hide either boniness or broadness by over-covering—drowning yourself in too much fabric.
3. Keeping your eye on the seam line—where it falls on your shoulder—to assess fit is a sure way to avoid mistakes.
4. Find the brands/designers that really fit your physique and design for your body type and always start there for your staples.

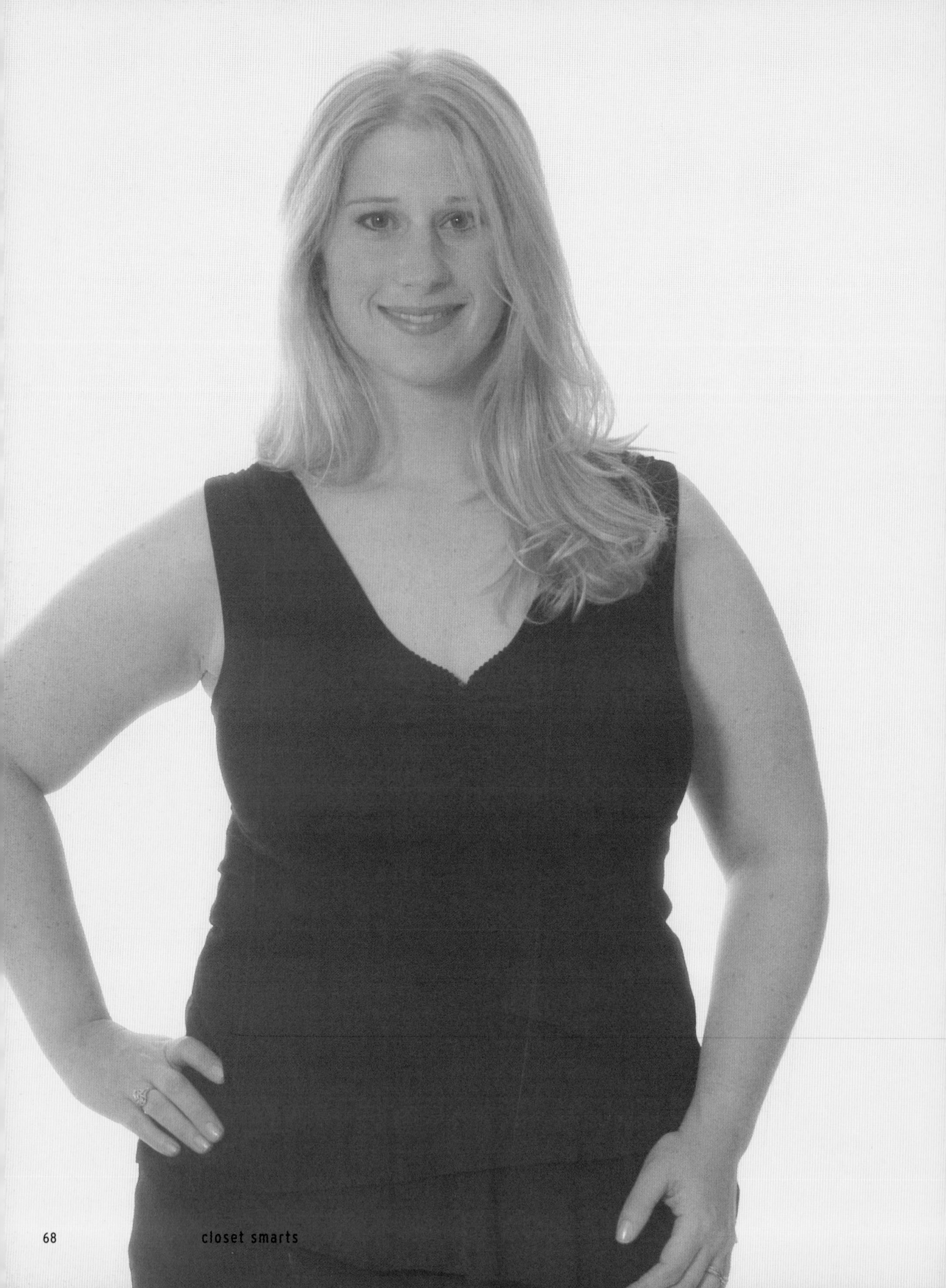

4

CHAPTER FOUR

dare to be bare!

Winning the Arms Race

In the previous chapter, we took a good hard look at shoulders as a largely overlooked, but serious, player in defining the silhouette of our upper halves. We got the first taste of just how we go about taking control of our silhouettes and shaping them more to our liking. In this chapter, we will cover another of the major building blocks of a good upper half: sleeve length. So roll up your sleeves, and let's show off our arms!

Arms Control

I've said this to you at the outset, and hopefully you have become reality-based enough at this point to go along with me: We are never all going to have nice little toned arms, free of waggle and cellulite and rough elbows, so if you are waiting (and waiting) to don short sleeves until your arms miraculously change their shape and become someone else's arms, stop now. Your arms are yours, and they're here to stay.

I say, let's find a way to make them look as good as they can. Let's focus on what we can change, not on what we wish would change. Even if you do start that arm-weight regimen you've been meaning to get to (how long have those free weights been staring at you from your bedroom floor?), you aren't going to change the basic shape of your arms. You may very well just have heavier arms genetically, and there's no changin' that! But there are good ways to show your arms without shame. As someone with heavy arms myself, I promise that it can be done tastefully rather than shamefully.

So what are the basic challenges? From what I have heard from our models and my other clients, there is the fear of fat arms (and the wag of flab), the fear of muscular arms (looking too bulky or tough), and the fear of scrawny arms (looking like you have sticks for limbs). Though in all cases, you can simply cover your arms as a basic strategy, I'd like to give you some tips on how to actually wear your arms bare, even if you feel sensitive about them. So here are three approaches. The common theme? Showing the entire arm turns out to be the best strategy for all three types of arm phobia. Why? Because when fabric cuts across the arm at any point, it draws attention to it.

Everyone really can *go sleeveless!*

If the heaviest part of your arm is the top half, you will not want to wear a cap sleeve, or a short sleeve that cuts across the middle of the upper section. Perhaps in your case, a three-quarter sleeve would be best. The same goes if you are muscular because chances are, the most buff/toned part of your arm is also that upper half. Any sleeve length that cuts across that portion of the arm will draw attention there. If your problem is boniness, though of course a bulkier-knit, longer-sleeved sweater would be a nice answer to add some girth, if you want to go bare, avoiding that fabric across the arm also improves your chances of minimizing the appearance of stick arms. Sleeves can look drapey or bell-like on a skinny arm unless they are super-fitted and proportionate.

If you've found a suitable blouse or shirt with flattering sleeves, go for it! But for a reliable strategy that works for all three types, look to the truly sleeveless. Now, let's take a look at how to do it best for all three types. We are going to use Lily, Felisha, and Deborah as our examples.

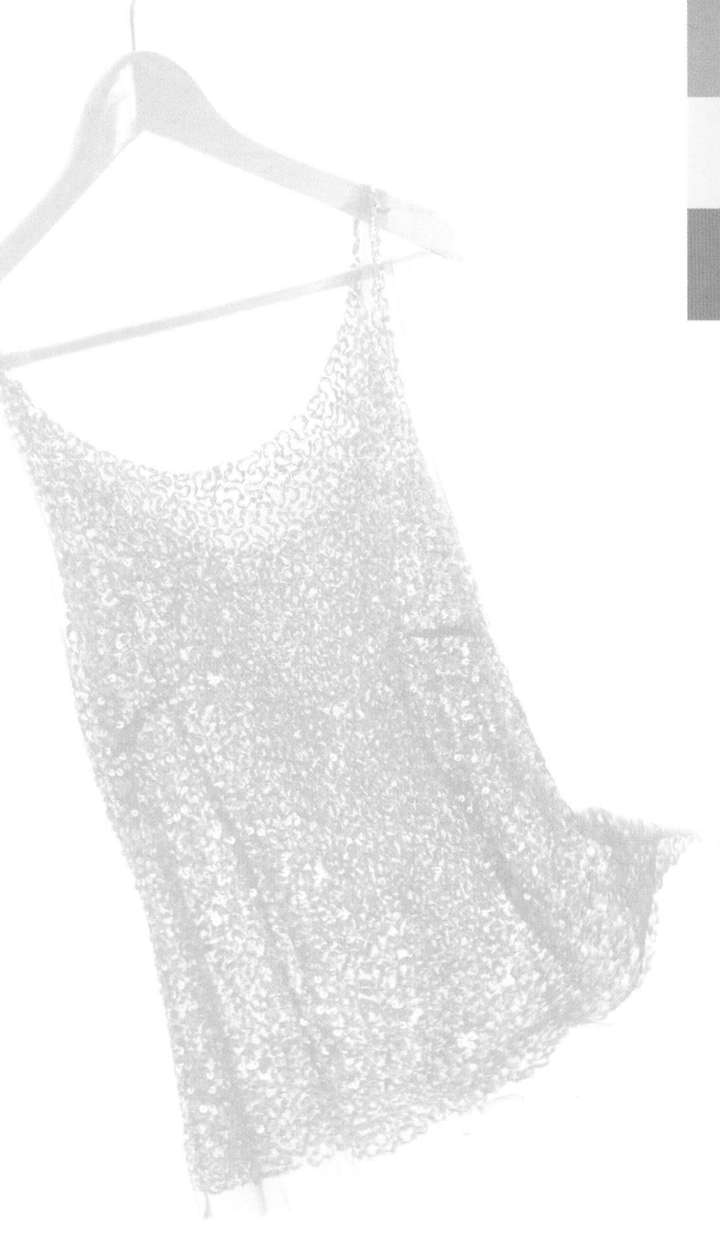

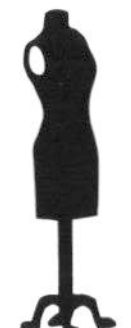

closet smarts:
HEAVY ARMS

HELPING OUT HEAVY ARMS

Lily is concerned about a lot of exposure for what she considers her heavy arms. Nonetheless, she likes to dress up and look sexy, and frankly, why should she always have to cover her arms up with a long sleeve, a shawl, or some other fashion accoutrement? When an arm is totally bare, as long as it is suitably surrounded by other design elements, it can truly blend right in to the whole package.

Bare arms can work for heavier arms too, as long as we don't draw attention to them

Our eyes are drawn to the good overall proportion of the outfit

lily now

In this photo, I have chosen to go **TRULY VOLUPTUOUS** with Lily, playing up her curves and **EXPOSING THE BEST PARTS** of her skin (her neckline, cleavage, ankle, and calf) to good effect. By choosing a stretch mesh empire top with thicker shoulder straps, Lily's smallest part is **HIGHLIGHTED** in the silhouette (the empire waist). Her bust shows off a **NICE CURVE** to match the curve of her hip, which is shown off by her mesh/stretch fluted skirt. The fluting at the bottom of the skirt in this case **BALANCES** out the accentuated hip and keeps the curvy look in proportion. In this overall silhouette, Lily's exposed arms fit right in and certainly do not attract a lot of attention as heavy. We simply aren't looking there, as there is nothing in the region to draw our eye to anything but the overall curvy silhouette. The places our eye is drawn are to the neck and bust, the cinch of the empire waist, and the ankle, as that is where the **LURE OF BARED SKIN** directs us to look.

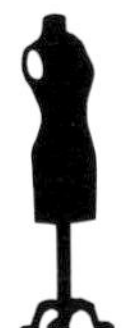

closet smarts: MUSCULAR ARMS

MAKING THE MOST OF MUSCULAR ARMS

Felisha brings us to our muscular arm query. She is broad-shouldered and generally a bit on the buff side on her upper half, but she doesn't like to appear that way when dressing. She is concerned to package her arms in a way that does not make them feel or look like salamis in their casings, even if they are toned salamis. Well, we are all prone to exaggeration when it comes to our bodily grievances, but let's take a look at a good strategy for downplaying the buff arm. Believe it or not, the halter is a great ally!

I am sure all this arm exposure feels counterintuitive to you, but listen (or look, as the case may be). It's really true. The reason the halter works so well on the buff arm is because it cuts away from the shoulder (usually the mother-load of bufficity), and thus away from the arm. By so doing the halter avoids cutting across and accentuating the areas of concern. (Buff arms are usually paired with broader shoulders.)

Muscular arms appear softer with a sloping shoulder and a sleeve that is not cut too close

felisha now

Here we see Felisha looking quite **LOVELY AND FEMININE** (if I may use the word to mean "softer-armed"). The main ploy, once again, is that our eye is not drawn to the arms themselves in looking at the overall silhouette. Rather, we are **FOCUSED ON THE NECKLINE AND DÉCOLLETAGE**, which become the real focal points because of a halter's cut. In addition, the halter adds the appearance of a squarer shoulder (where Felisha's are quite round and broad), as its line is cut diagonally across the chest and upper body. So she gets two silhouette fixes for the price of one!

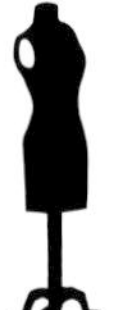

closet smarts:
BONY ARMS

BALANCING BONY ARMS

And what about the bony-armed, you ask? Here we turn to Deborah for instruction. We saw her in the past chapter dealing with bony shoulders, and in the case of her arms, the same tricks apply.

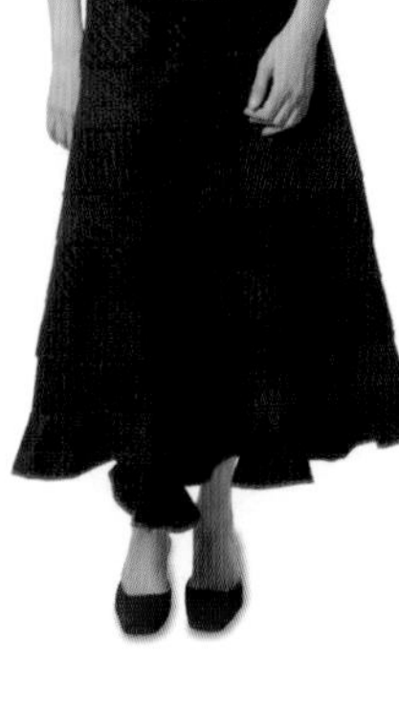

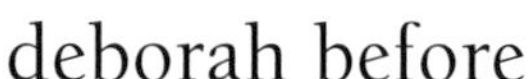

A skinny strap emphasizes a skinny arm

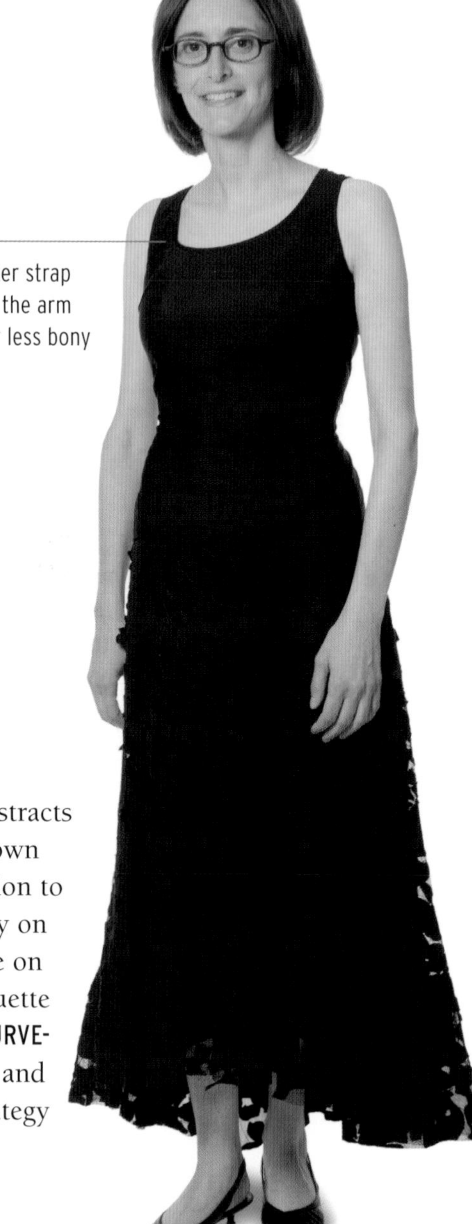

A thicker strap makes the arm appear less bony

deborah before

Here we see spaghetti straps overemphasizing the slenderness of Deborah's shoulders and arms, making them look even more frail and sticklike as they echo the shape of the thin straps.

deborah now

See how something as simple as a **THICKER STRAP** distracts the eye from the appearance of thinness. Toning down the angle of the shoulder really **SOFTENS** the transition to the arm. Since there is no fabric falling immediately on the arm to give us any real comparative perspective on its width, we are led to the rest of the outfit's silhouette to guide us—in this case, a **FIGURE-HUGGING** (and **CURVE-ENHANCING**) top and a fuller bottom that adds girth and shape to Deborah's bottom half as well (a good strategy overall for the thin amongst us).

4

The Last Word

So you see, everyone really *can* go sleeveless! Stop hiding your arms away and over-covering as your only option for dealing with arm insecurities. The truth is, we could all spend the rest of our lives over-covering as an answer to many of our figure insecurities, but it is *not* our only option, and it is often not the best one. In many instances, it just brings out the flaws we're trying to hide. A better solution, as counterintuitive as it may be to your inner fear–driven fashion instincts, is always to show *more*. The psychological pivot here is taking control of your silhouette—or just realizing that you *can* take control of it.

In the next chapter, we'll discuss some handy tricks of design that help mask trouble spots in the belly zone through design innovations, fabric variation, and styling. These tricks of the trade can help shape and mask your silhouette to your heart's content.

ULTIMATE ARMS STYLE

Whether your arms are toned and muscled, skinny, heavy, or wobbly, they'll look much more attractive with these style tips.

1. Bare is beautiful when it comes to arms!
2. If your sleeves cut across a problem area, they'll draw attention to it.
3. Choose the strap width that works with your arms: slimmer straps for bigger arms, wider straps for thinner arms.
4. Distraction, distraction! Use your décolletage and other enticing areas to draw attention away from less-than-perfect arms.

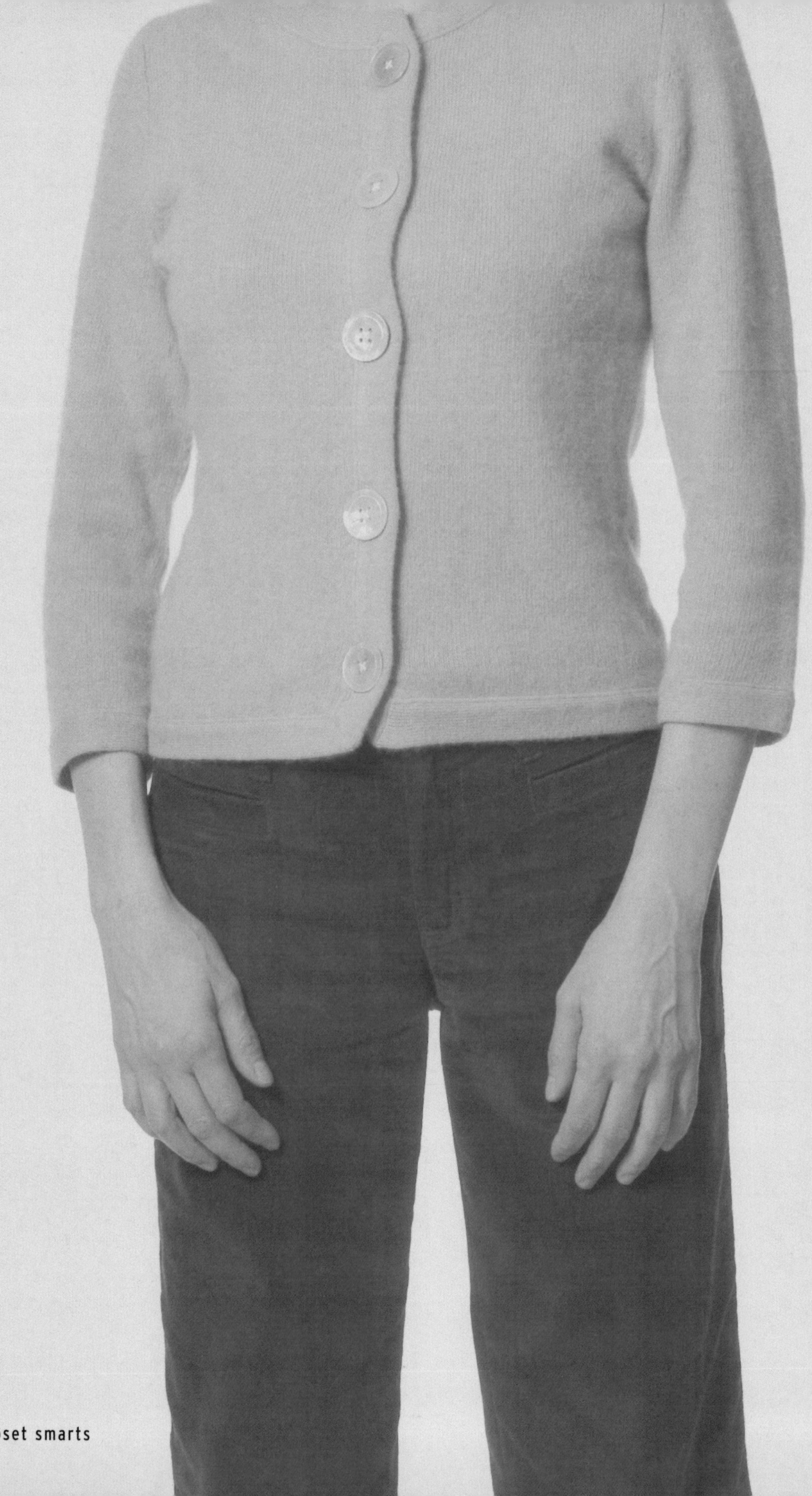

CHAPTER FIVE

the fits of your knits

And Other Great Tales of Design

5

In this last chapter on the upper half, I want to show you a few no-fail ways to deal with the overall project of reshaping your top half. If I haven't convinced you that jackets are one of the best ways to achieve this effect, well, at least you have this chapter to fall back on. If you are concerned about a tummy, you'll also really get some help here, with tips on masking those extra rolls and drawing the eye to other, slimmer parts of your torso. And, of course, there's always that décolletage to focus in on.

Sweaters: The Good, the Bad, and the Ugly

I already covered a little bit about sweaters in chapter 2, when I took on the tragedy of the turtleneck. My drift there? Very basically, it's really not a great idea to add a bunch of girth to your frame with a bulky sweater, at least as far as most of us are concerned. (Skinny Minnies or tall ladies have more leeway.) In the less-bulky sweater department, however, a different idea applies: A sweater, utilitarian as it ostensibly may be, is in fact an *opportunity* to add shape and style to your overall look—so don't miss it!

CARDIGANS: THE OLD STANDBY

Probably the most depressing, or should I say, *boring*, example of sweater dressing is the monochromatic cardigan set, especially when it involves a turtleneck. Remember Sara?

Though some might consider a monochromatic sweater set, turtleneck or no, a classic look, in my book, it's a missed opportunity. It's boring, for the most part usually shapeless, and does no real work for an outfit. It's more like settling for something that appears to be an outfit, but is really just a stopgap measure, a poor excuse for fashion coordination. They also tend to be crewnecked, and you know how I feel about that! If you are a cardiganaholic (and you know who you are), do me a favor and at least pair your endless collection of limp and lifeless, drab-colored cover-ups with an exciting camisole or a really formfitting and richly colored layering garment. Please? Otherwise, you might try an alternative in the same genre, something like this form-hugging sweater jacket as seen on Lily (next page).

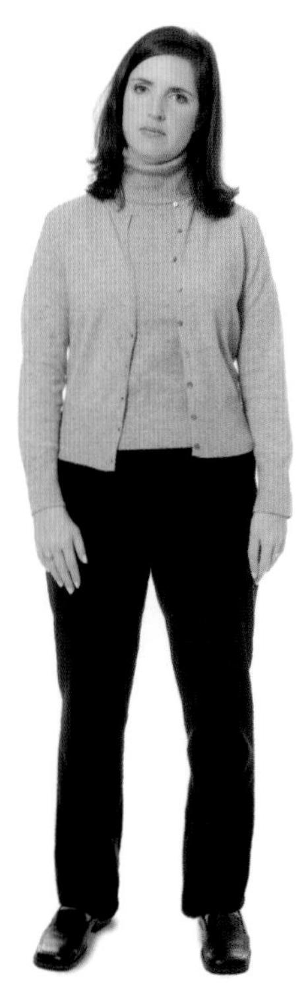

bad cardigan

Here's Sara in her monochromatic sweater set. Ugh! Truly sad.

5

A sweater is an opportunity to add shape and style to your look.

Open neck draws the eye here

A nice overall shape enhanced with the wonders of Lycra!

Arm coverage for the cold or fearful

We see a waist!

A scalloped hem eases over her hips, creating a great shape

good cardigan

In essence, Lily's sweater gives the same feel as a cardigan without the inherent boxiness of it, while providing a **GREAT V-NECK** and an excellent **CURVY SHAPE** through Lily's top half. The cotton and Lycra mix have enough **STRUCTURE** to really smooth out any potential bumps in this area and provide **GOOD TUMMY COVERAGE**. This sweater **DRAWS THE EYE** to all the right places as it cinches at the empire waist, keeps the neck open, and scallops away at the bottom, **FLATTERING THE HIPS**. And it reveals some nice color layering—another means of creating and controlling your silhouette.

closet smarts:
RESHAPING WITH SWEATERS

CLOSET SMARTS STYLE: SWEATERS WITH SASS

The sweaterlette (a.k.a bolero sweater) in all its many forms can perform many functions for us, from shaping the silhouette—including covering arms, giving shoulders more structure, and cinching in our narrowest part—to adding that little bit of sass to an otherwise humdrum outfit with sequins, embroidery, or a splash of color.

One caveat about this sweater shape, however, is to watch out where it cuts on your chest. There are as many different cuts as there are sweaters, and you really need to try them on to make sure you end up with one that doesn't cut you in an awkward spot.

Everyone's top halves are different, and obviously, most clothing is not made to fit every shape and size. Look for one that just brushes the sides of your bust or nicely covers your boobs and drapes well below them. Avoid those that cut right across your bust or that have extra folds of fabric hanging around under your boobs—no good. Every part of the sweater should be meaningfully utilized to enhance your shape.

Here are two great cardigan looks for Beth, whom we might call our classic pear.

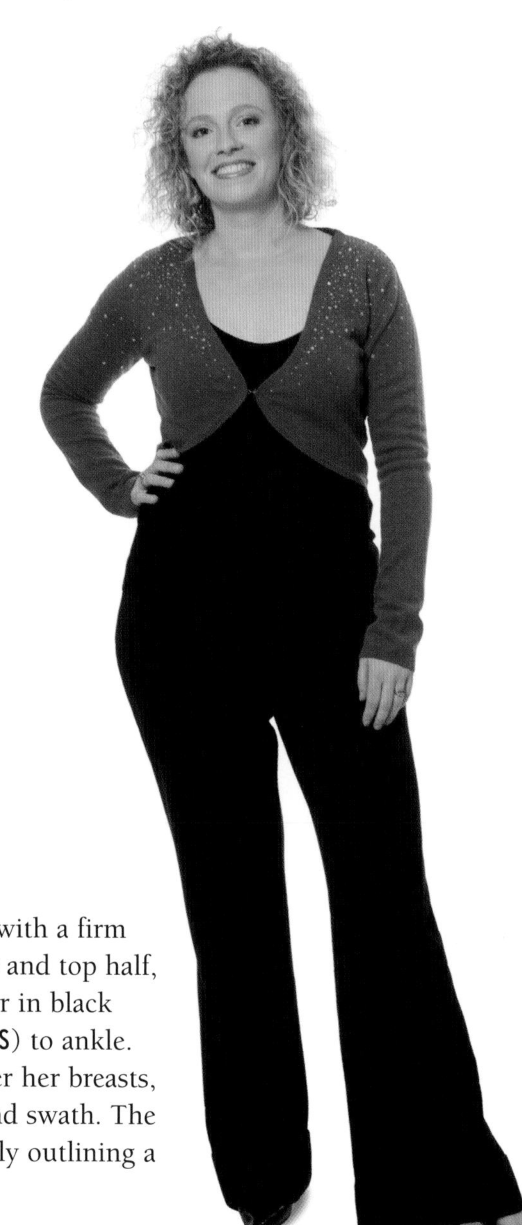

beth now

In this first picture, we use the bolero sweater with a firm layering piece to **ACCENT** Beth's petite shoulders and top half, while **SMOOTHING OUT HER BELLY** and clothing her in black from torso (including, of course, her **CURVY HIPS**) to ankle. The bolero provides good smooth coverage over her breasts, while **ENHANCING THEIR SHAPE** through its cut and swath. The sweater's shape hugs Beth's narrowest part, really outlining a nice shape and line for her midsection.

In this next sweater look, we see the beauty of the *unconventional* cardigan set. Here is one that really works the torso to its best advantage!

Open neck and embroidered detail draw the eye here.

beth now

The camisole is very delicate at the top where Beth is smallest (you can't see it all, but there are spaghetti straps), and flares into an A-line at the hip, where Beth's silhouette tends to be wider, flowing out over the curve of her hips for a **SMOOTHER LINE** at midsection. The cardigan repeats this shape as it flares out just above the hip, actually making her hips look *narrower* than they are and adding a bit more substance to her narrow shoulders to keep everything in **BALANCE**. In addition, look at all the **ADORABLE DESIGN DETAILS** this set adds to Beth's overall **SENSE OF STYLE**—the embroidery, the satin piping, and the gorgeous deep wine color. Now, *this* is a sweater set I can really get behind!

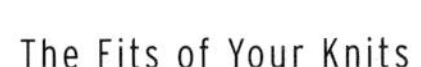

Let's take a look at Amy next. She is a huge fan of cardigans, but like most people, she wore them more as a fallback option—something that was easy to throw on and "match" with things. Of course, that's exactly what they ended up looking like—or worse, like a utilitarian choice for warmth's sake. Can you say it with me? Missed opportunity…

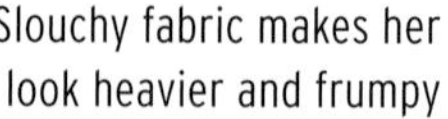

Slouchy fabric makes her
look heavier and frumpy

amy before

Despite the nicer scoop of Amy's layered top, this cardigan literally seems to pull her boobs down her chest, and it generally adds a feel of sagging frumpiness to her overall look. Why, I say? It doesn't have to be this way! A sweater has to be doing more than simply adding girth to your silhouette to justify wearing it. If it's not fitted, it should be a sweater coat, and if it's a sweater coat, unless you are 5'7" or above, it should still be very lightweight and slim-fitting rather than bulky.

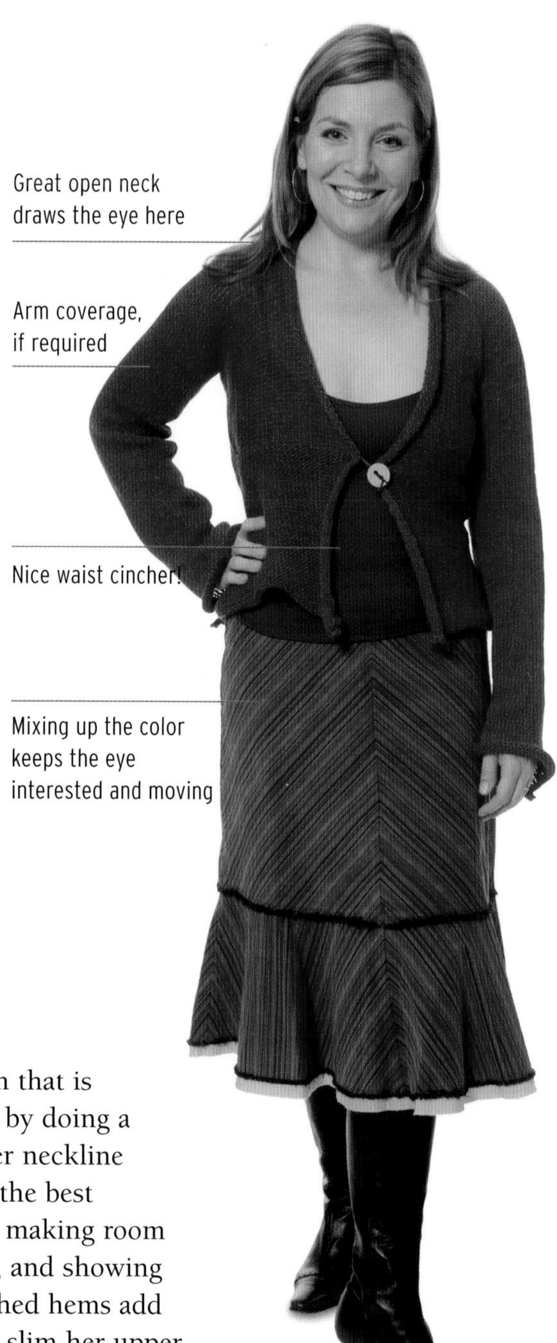
Great open neck draws the eye here
Arm coverage, if required
Nice waist cincher!
Mixing up the color keeps the eye interested and moving

amy now

Now, here's the perfect example of a cardigan that is actually earning its place in Amy's wardrobe by doing a little **WORK FOR HER FIGURE**: While keeping her neckline open, this sweater **CINCHES AMY'S WAIST** in at the best possible spot and falls away in **A NICE A-LINE**, making room for her hips, enhancing her hourglass shape, and showing some **EXCITING COLOR** underneath. Its unfinished hems add an arty bit of personality, and its bell sleeves slim her upper arms. What isn't this sweater doing for Amy's shape? It may as well have been sewn on her!

For Karen, whose shape tends to be a bit boxy, we tried a formfitting sweater.

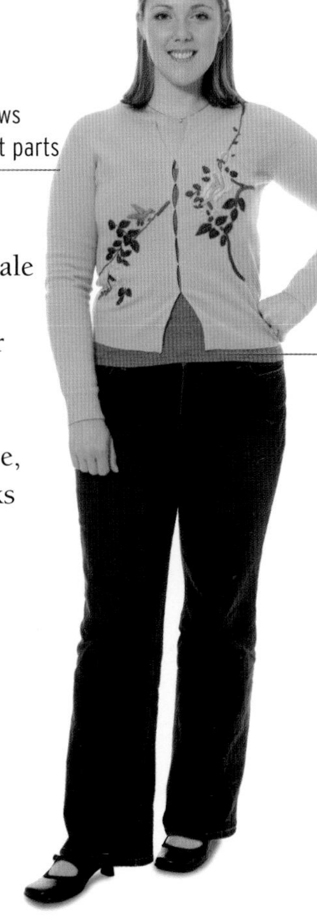
Form fit shows
her slimmest parts
Bright colors
add interest
and dimension

karen now

Karen's **FORMFITTING** sweater has a hook-and-eye-closure in pale green with great embroidered detail, accented with a darker pink layering piece beneath. You have to admit, this is better than any old sweater set. This sweater, while helping us see a nice upper shape on Karen, also has **LOADS OF PERSONALITY AND STYLE**, and it really gives Karen the opportunity, stylewise, to make a statement in that regard. We left the last few hooks undone to accentuate the appearance of the waist and make the hips' curve contribute to more like an hourglass, rather than square, silhouette. This, too, is the kind of cardigan I could get excited about.

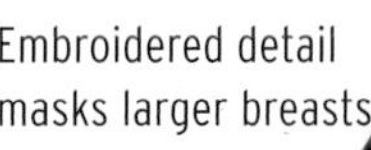
Embroidered detail
masks larger breasts
Shortened waist

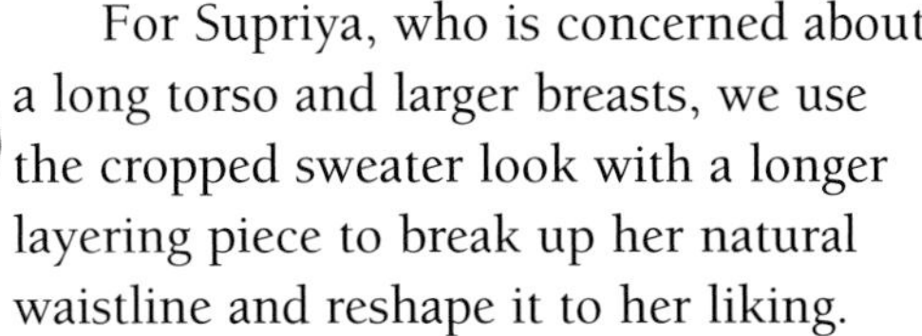

For Supriya, who is concerned about a long torso and larger breasts, we use the cropped sweater look with a longer layering piece to break up her natural waistline and reshape it to her liking.

supriya now

This cardigan cuts Supriya where a natural waist might be, and combined with a long Lycra top beneath and lower-waisted pants, it completely **RESHAPES HER UPPER HALF** to her own liking. The tuxedo-type beaded embroidery is a great topper to the men's-cut pant, but paired with red heels keeps the whole look **FEMININE AND SHARP**. Can you believe how versatile these cardigans can be? Who knew?

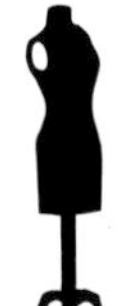

closet smarts:
SWEATERS FOR STRUCTURE

Where Deborah, our skinny Minnie, is concerned, we chose a cardigan with some boxiness to it, to add a bit more structure to her narrow upper half.

Open neck draws the eye here

Fitted camisole beneath reminds us that she has a flat tummy and boobs!

Some girth is added at the waist without looking overwhelmed in fabric

deborah now

Playing with a palette of warm browns, we used texture and small details, like the beaded piping on this sweater, to create a **DISTINCTIVE LOOK** for Deborah. The Lycra satin camisole shows her shape, so that the boxier wool cardigan can afford to be boxy without turning her into a box! Meanwhile, its boxier shape helps add some much-needed substance to Deborah's top half to keep her from looking overly skinny. Because her camisole has a **NICE DEEP SCOOP**, keeping **HER NECK WIDE OPEN, THE HIGHER CREW NECK** on the sweater doesn't close her up, but rather adds an **INTERESTING ARCHITECTURAL FEATURE** to her décolletage, and we leave it open for this reason.

Deborah's darker side?

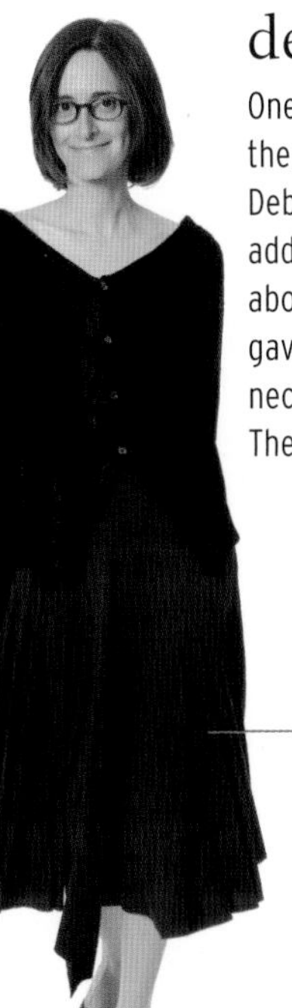

deborah before

One look should be enough for you to see that there is way too much fabric here to be doing Deborah's frame any good. This is not the way to add more substance to a small frame. Everything about this velvet cardigan that Deborah thought gave her a graceful, flowy look is too big—the V-neck, the shoulder seams, the width—she is lost. The top has won. It is wearing her. Not good!

Deborah is swimming in this!

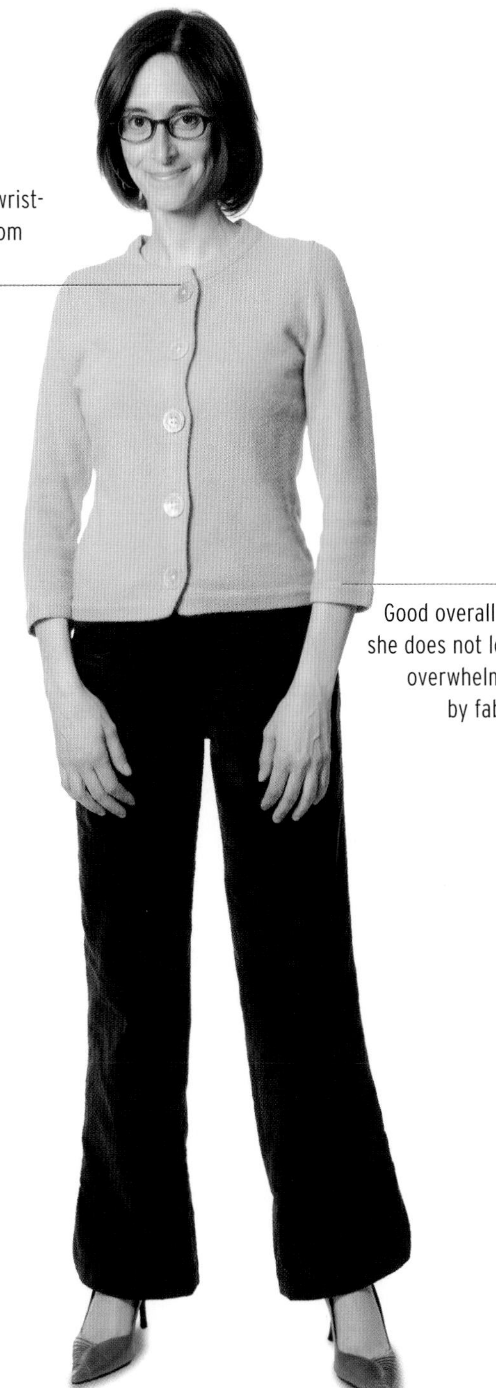

Big buttons and wrist-bands distract from her thinness

Good overall fit, she does not look overwhelmed by fabric

Another great cardigan look for Deborah? A thicker bouclé sweater jacket.

deborah now

Though small enough to **FIT HER FIGURE** well, the wide-banded details—of the crew neck, waistband, button placket, and sleeves—as well as the large-scale buttons, achieve the effect of giving Deborah more substance and width, despite her very narrow frame. Because of the **FORMFITTING** nature of this sweater jacket, we get to see the curve of Deborah's bust, as well as some **DEFINITION OF A WAIST**. She is as **SHAPELY AS THEY COME** in this great sweater, another topper which is really earning its place in her wardrobe as it (re)works her figure to highlight its best assets.

closet smarts:
SWEATER ACCENTS

On our tallest model, Morgan, we tried two looks, the first of which is a layered cardigan effect.

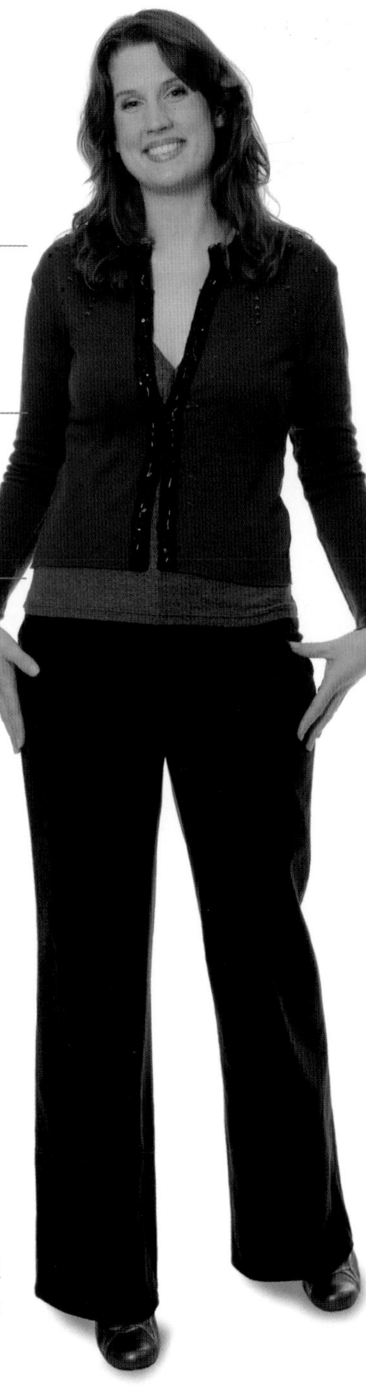

Sparkly placket adds pizzazz to the open neckline

Empire closure adds a cinch in the right place

Layering with color helps smooth over and distract from the tummy

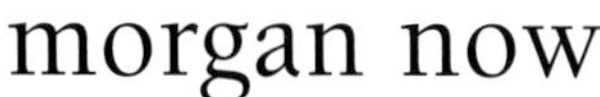

morgan now

Here we use several design tricks to achieve the desired effect—a smooth-looking midsection—by keeping the eye moving. First, we mix up the color palette with a variety of neutrals that blend well, but are unexpected in combination. Next, we close the cardigan at a narrow place on Morgan's torso (the empire waist). In constructing her neckline (remember, we're in charge), we mix her V-neck Lycra top with a higher, but open, crewnecked cardigan, drawing the eye ever upward to her **GORGEOUS FACE**. As for her torso, in keeping the length of the Lycra top longer than the sweater (the layering effect), the eye travels down from her **LOVELY DÉCOLLETAGE** to her long legs, further enhanced by the vertical beading detail that runs along the button placket. All of these elements help achieve the appearance of a **LONG, SLEEK TORSO**. The cardigan itself is made of a fine-gauge merino wool, so there is no bulking effect despite the added layer. So many tricks going on, are you paying attention?

For Morgan's next look, we use some of the same tricks and some new ones.

morgan now

The gauge of Morgan's sweater is a finer cotton (so no bulk), and it cinches at the empire waist (the **NARROWEST PART** of the silhouette). Using it with the deep V-neck and the lighter-colored print and **FORMFITTING STYLE** of the top, we create a **VERY SLIM**-looking combination for Morgan. As the A-line cut of the sweater flares out over her hips, we also enhance the appearance of those **NEVER-ENDING LEGS**. So our eye is drawn to her face and neck, travels to her empire waist, and then down to her long legs. What could be better? She looks absolutely **SVELTE AND FABULOUS**!

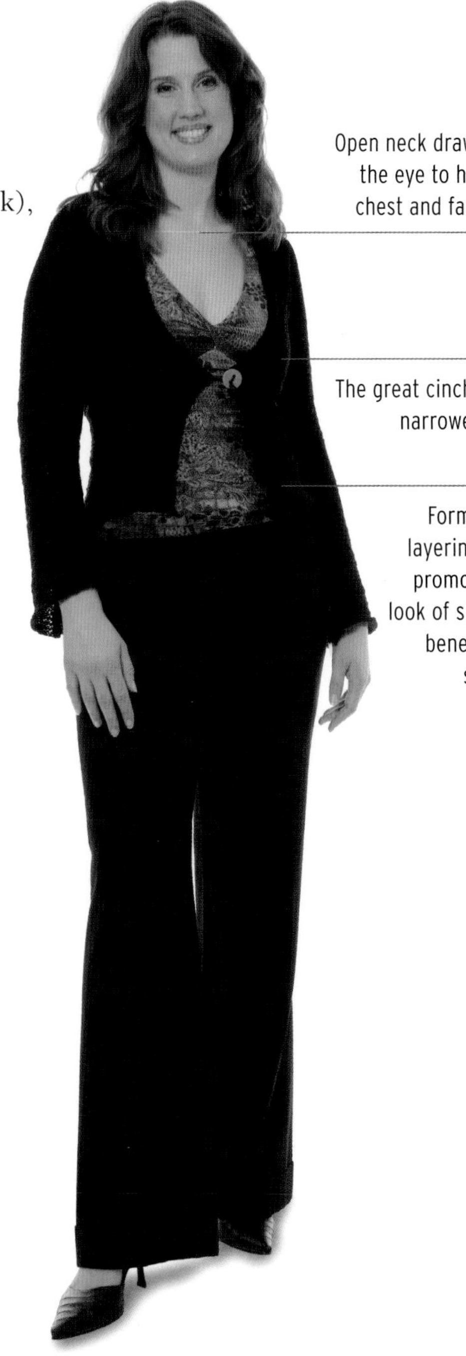

Open neck draws the eye to her chest and face

The great cinch at the narrowest part

Form fitting layering piece promotes the look of slimness beneath the sweater

So what have you learned about cardigans and their layering friends here? A good fit is always the first place to start. Then work to minimize or disguise your obvious figure problems and to accent the best parts of your torso with the various shape-sculpters we have seen so far in this chapter: crop, shape, sleeve length, placket size and style, closures, decorative detail, etc. You have many options, so there is no reason to use the cardigan set as a simple and easy alternative to actually *thinking* about your outfit. It is a dangerous myth that such a set always looks good. So right now, start remaking this old habit by pulling apart all of the sets you already own and try wearing them in combination with other things—camisoles, longer tops for layering, different colors, and even printed tops! Just get rid of the turtlenecks, that's all I ask.

OTHER SWEATER MATTERS: TRICKS OF THE TRADE

We covered a lot with our cardigan explorations in terms of basic sweater dressing and the art of dressing and *ad*dressing your midsection, but let's take a closer look at some of the strategies we got a peek at earlier. When you want to upgrade your look and appear more put-together and polished, avoid bulky knit tops (mostly commonly found in the sweater department). Go for the skinny sweater instead!

Some good examples? Let's see what our models can show you.

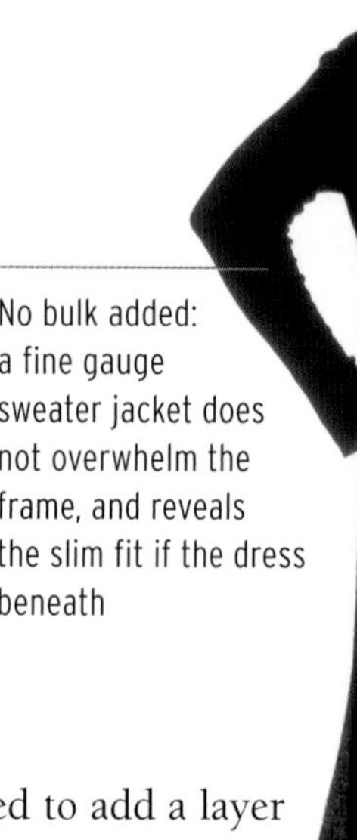

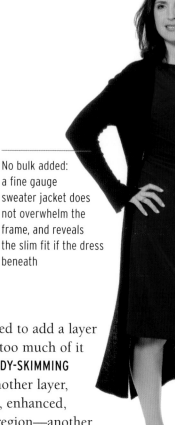

No bulk added: a fine gauge sweater jacket does not overwhelm the frame, and reveals the slim fit if the dress beneath

sara now

Sara, who claims she is always chilly, wanted to add a layer over her **SEXY RED DRESS**. Rather than hide too much of it with a jacket or cardigan, we chose this **BODY-SKIMMING** thin-knit sweater jacket. This gives Sara another layer, but it still shows her **GREAT FIGURE** beneath, enhanced, of course, by the shirring across the belly region—another great device for shaping the figure to your liking.

supriya now

Here is Surpriya in a sweater with an elasticized waist. With its **REFINED** knit, this sweater serves to really **UPGRADE** her look (to **UPSCALE CASUAL** vis-à-vis her dark denim jeans), and, with its waist detail, the sweater helps mask her longer torso.

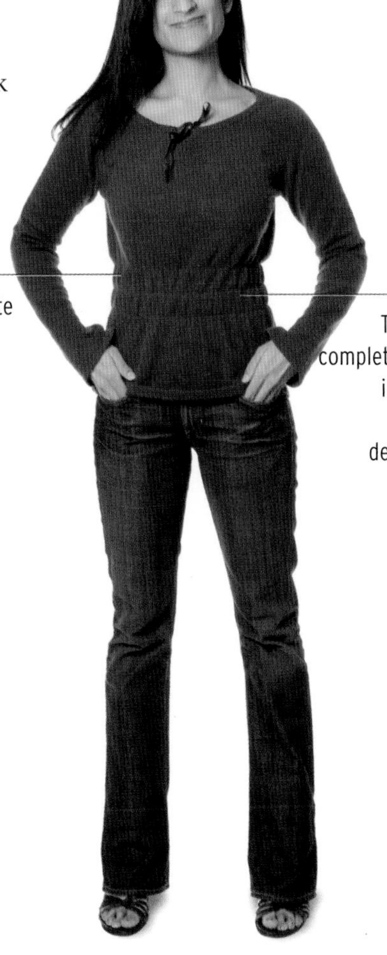

We recreate her waist where she wants it

This sweater completes an outfit in itself with interesting design details

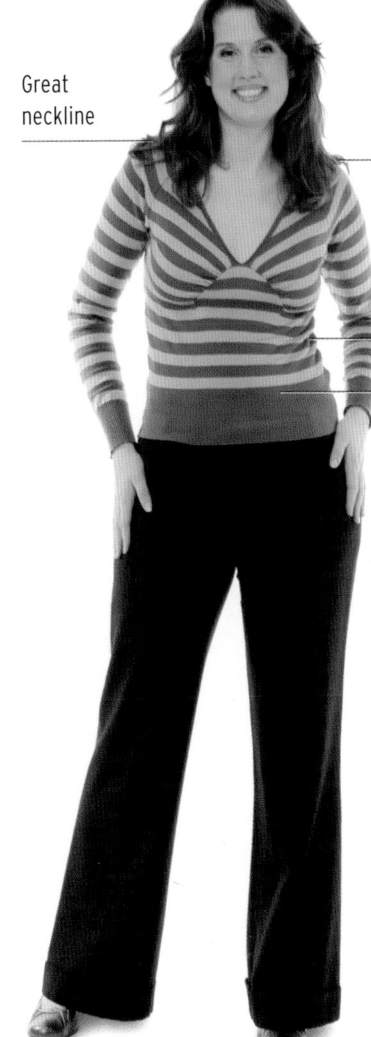

Great neckline

Outfit topper: who needs layers with this great number?

Form fit creates waist and smoothes over tummy

Wide waistband smoothes over hips

morgan now

Here's Morgan in a great fine-knit, horizontal-stripe sweater that adds **CLASS AND SASS** to her tall stature. The variation in the stripe around her boobs adds **DIMENSION** and distraction, drawing the eye, again, toward her **DÉCOLLETAGE** and taking some of the wind out of the old mantra that horizontal stripes always do a disservice to your figure. With Morgan's lower-waisted and wide-legged trouser, her overall appearance is smooth and **CHIC**, and the look is extremely **FIGURE-FLATTERING**.

closet smarts:
SEXY SWEATERS

CLOSET SMARTS STYLE: SHAPELY SWEATERS

The figure-hugging sweaters in this section are the sort you should be homing in on. They function as outfit-toppers in and of themselves, even as they provide more warmth than the average cotton top. They should be fitted to your body, working for your figure, and integrated into your overall look rather than used simply as a layer for extra warmth. They can be combined with other tops that help obscure problem torsos in all sorts of ways, as you can see from the photos on these pages.

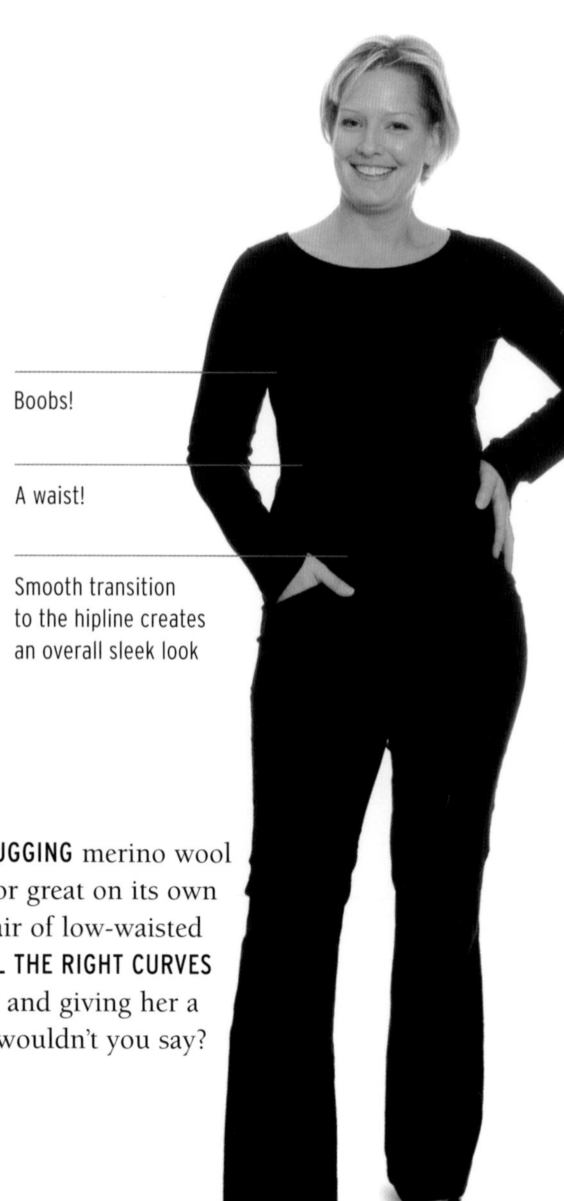

Boobs!

A waist!

Smooth transition to the hipline creates an overall sleek look

felisha now

And here's Felisha in a **FINE-GAUGE, FIGURE-HUGGING** merino wool sweater, suitable for **LAYERING** with a jacket or great on its own as shown here. Paired with a sleek-fitting pair of low-waisted stretch pants, this ensemble **ACCENTUATES ALL THE RIGHT CURVES** for Felisha, **SLIMMING** over the rougher spots and giving her a **CLASSY AND POLISHED** sweater-dressing look, wouldn't you say?

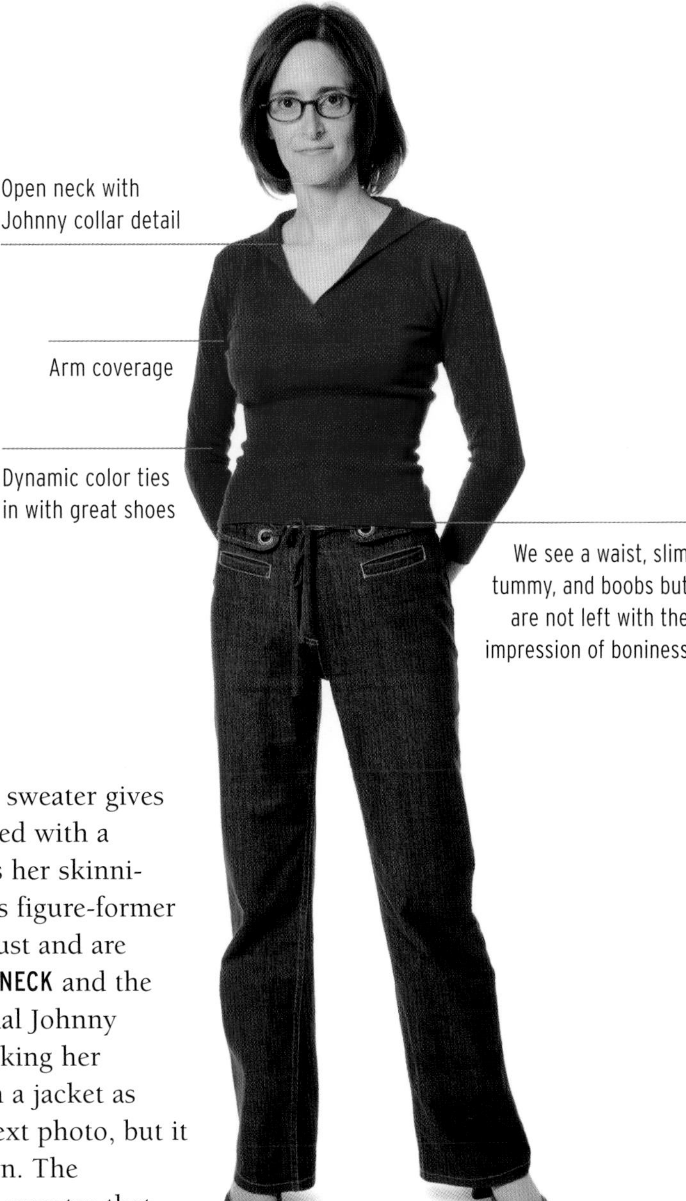

deborah now

Look at the **SEXY CURVES** this **FORMFITTING** sweater gives to our skinny Minnie, Deborah! Combined with a wider-legged dark denim jean that masks her skinniness, Deborah gets all the **BENEFITS** of this figure-former and none of its drawbacks. We see her bust and are drawn to her **DÉCOLLETAGE** via the **DEEP V-NECK** and the **DRAMATIC** wine color, even as its traditional Johnny collar adds structure to her top half, masking her boniness. She could easily layer this with a jacket as well to good effect, as you'll see in the next photo, but it is very **FLATTERING** to her figure on its own. The finer-gauge wool adds a **SLEEKNESS** to the sweater that gives her overall outfit, even paired with jeans, an **UPSCALE CASUAL** effect.

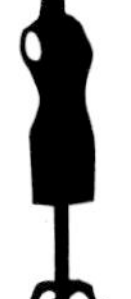

closet smarts: SWEATER COMBOS

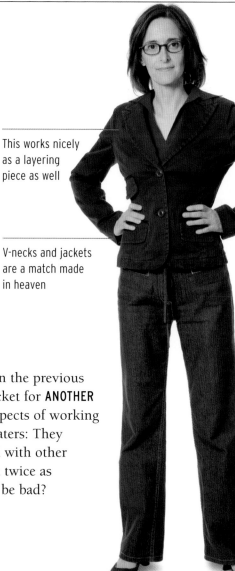

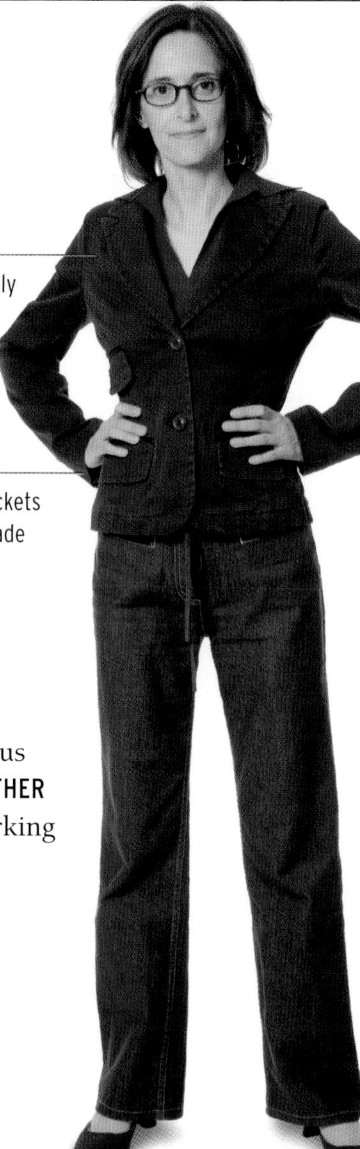

This works nicely as a layering piece as well

V-necks and jackets are a match made in heaven

deborah now

Here is Deborah in the same sweater as in the previous photo, but this time, it's paired with a jacket for **ANOTHER GREAT LOOK**. That is one of the greatest aspects of working with "skinnier" (read **MORE REFINED**) sweaters: They can both stand alone, as well as pair well with other pieces without bulking up. That's at least twice as many outfits per sweater... how can that be bad?

Use sweaters as layering devices with formfitting tops to create interesting combinations.

deborah now

Another sweater look for Deborah that adds a little more substance to her slight frame is this empire tie-back (or front, as the case may be) gray wool number. The **FULLER-BODIED** shape of this sweater adds some width to Deborah even as the empire tie allows her to create some **SHAPE** through her torso, so she doesn't appear overwhelmed in fabric. (She is also aided by the finer-gauge wool to avoid the "Help! I'm drowning in my sweater" look.) Its A-line drape combined with a wide-legged trouser also adds some substance to Deborah's frame while giving a **SOPHISTICATED AND CLASSIC LINE** to her overall silhouette.

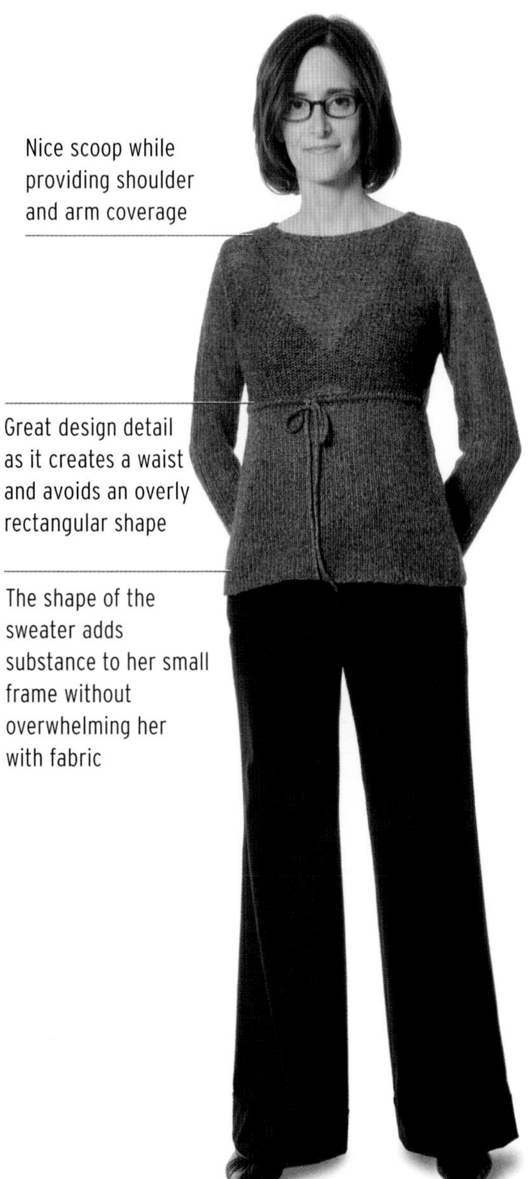

Nice scoop while providing shoulder and arm coverage

Great design detail as it creates a waist and avoids an overly rectangular shape

The shape of the sweater adds substance to her small frame without overwhelming her with fabric

So you see, sweater dressing doesn't have to mean dressing down for the sake of warmth! Stick to refined sweaters that actually work *with* your wardrobe—sweaters that *add* something to your outfits. The best way to go is to stick with finer-gauge (less bulky) knits and sweaters that have some design details built in, just as any other tops would have (darts; interesting closures, cut, and necklines; and even embroidered details). Use sweaters as layering devices with formfitting tops to create interesting combinations that can draw the eye toward good areas and away from the bad ones on your top half. And use strategies like shirring, cinching, texture, and print in that layering mix to further enforce your silhouette-shaping strategies.

closet smarts:
WRAPS FOR WIDER HIPS

The Wrap Top and the Empire Waist: Looks for Every Body

Last but not least, when it comes to your upper half and reshaping your torso, the wrap top and the empire waist are two styles I have found it hard to make anybody look bad in. This is great news! When you see an empire waist or a wrap top (faux or no), at least give it a try. It's much more likely to look good on you than many other styles.

The empire waist works because, as I have said repeatedly throughout this book, it is simply the narrowest part of everyone's frame—what could be bad about that? One potential drawback: If the fit is too loose, it can make you look pregnant, which is bad, unless you are pregnant, so do watch out for that. There are plenty of empire styles that are shaped through the bodice to varying degrees so that you can mask to your heart's content in the tummy department.

The wrap top is great, too: first, because it tends to wrap around the empire waist (narrow), but also because it totally showcases your décolletage—lovely! Again, what could be better? Here are just a few broad-ranging examples as showcased by our models. Check them out, and you'll see what wrap tops and empire waists can do for your figure!

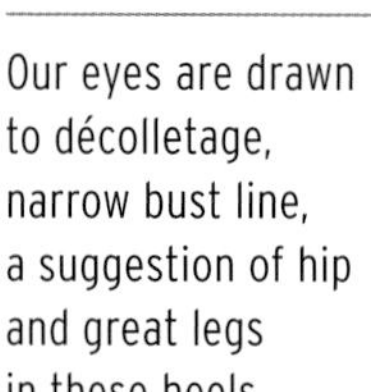
Our eyes are drawn to décolletage, narrow bust line, a suggestion of hip and great legs in these heels

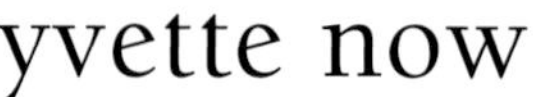
yvette now

Yvette models a wrap dress that's **PERFECT** for showing a **SHAPELY CHEST** while concealing it tastefully and **DRAPING NICELY** away from below the bust (the empire waist) to conceal problem areas in the belly and hips.

CLOSET SMARTS STYLE: UNDER WRAPS

The wrap dress is a real winner on almost any figure. Diane von Furstenberg perfected this look, and though her dresses are certainly more expensive than most, luckily for us, there have been many knock-offs since.

Try a wrap dress and see the wonders it can do for your figure. If you are more troubled through the tummy area, look for a patterned version, like the swirly fabric on Yvette's dress on page 94. A print adds an extra element of camouflage, distracting the eye from potential problems. Look for fabrics that drape well over the body (rather than cling), or for fabrics that have more substance so as to smooth over lumps and bumps.

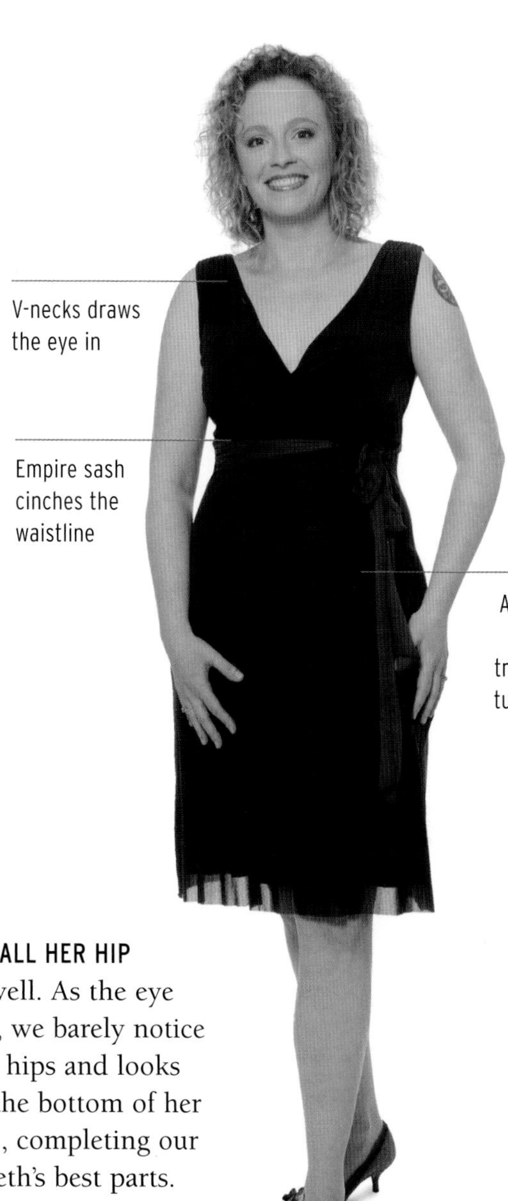

V-necks draws the eye in

Empire sash cinches the waistline

A-line drape covers her troublesome tummy, hips, and rear

beth now

Here is Beth in an empire-waisted dress that **SOLVES ALL HER HIP PROBLEMS** and smoothes nicely over her tummy as well. As the eye is drawn to her dress's sash and the **LOVELY NECKLINE**, we barely notice what falls below except that it flows nicely over her hips and looks **VERY FEMININE**. With a **REFINED HEEL** in flashy red at the bottom of her ensemble, our eye is also drawn to her **SHAPELY CALF**, completing our camouflage strategy by keeping our eyes on all of Beth's best parts.

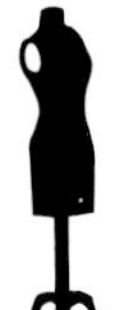

closet smarts:
SHAPELY WRAPS

beth now

WRAP TOPS work well with pants, too. Beth, here, dons an empire-waisted faux wrap top that **DOES WONDERS** to conceal the tummy area and work around her hips. The scalloped shape of the top's hem also **FLOWS NICELY** over the hips to keep a **SMOOTH STREAMLINED APPEARANCE**, elongating the look of Beth's legs as well.

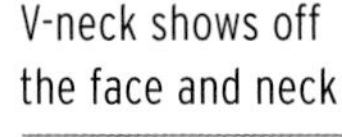

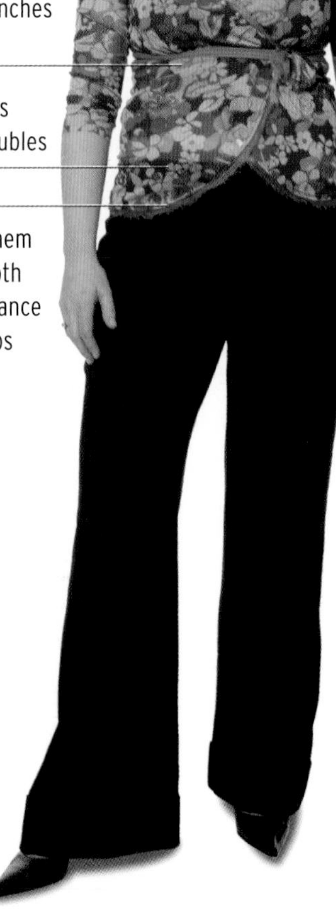

Empire cinches her waist

Wrap masks tummy troubles

Scalloped hem helps smooth the appearance of large hips

V-neck draws eye in

Top gives nice accentuation of her bust

Thick waistband smoothes over her hips

amy now

Amy also models a faux wrap dress to good effect. Here we see another common design strategy that often comes along with the wrap dress or top—*shirring*. We've seen this before, and it's a great way to **MASK POTENTIAL PROBLEMS** in the tummy region. The purposely drapey fall of the fabric allows for a little give in the bumps and rolls department, while maintaining the **SLEEK SILHOUETTE** of a closer-fitting garment. Do I need to say anything about **HOW GREAT AMY LOOKS** here? I think you can see for yourself how this works.

amy now

Here's another example of a wrap dress. This one uses a **BOLD PATTERN** in addition to its shape to **ENHANCE** Amy's figure. As you can see, a wrap that **HIGHLIGHTS** the empire waist, opens up the neck, and drapes nicely over the hips is **A WINNER** on many levels. This **BOLD** striped dress also has **A LOT OF STYLE** to it and looks fab with Amy's tall brown leather boots. She looks great!

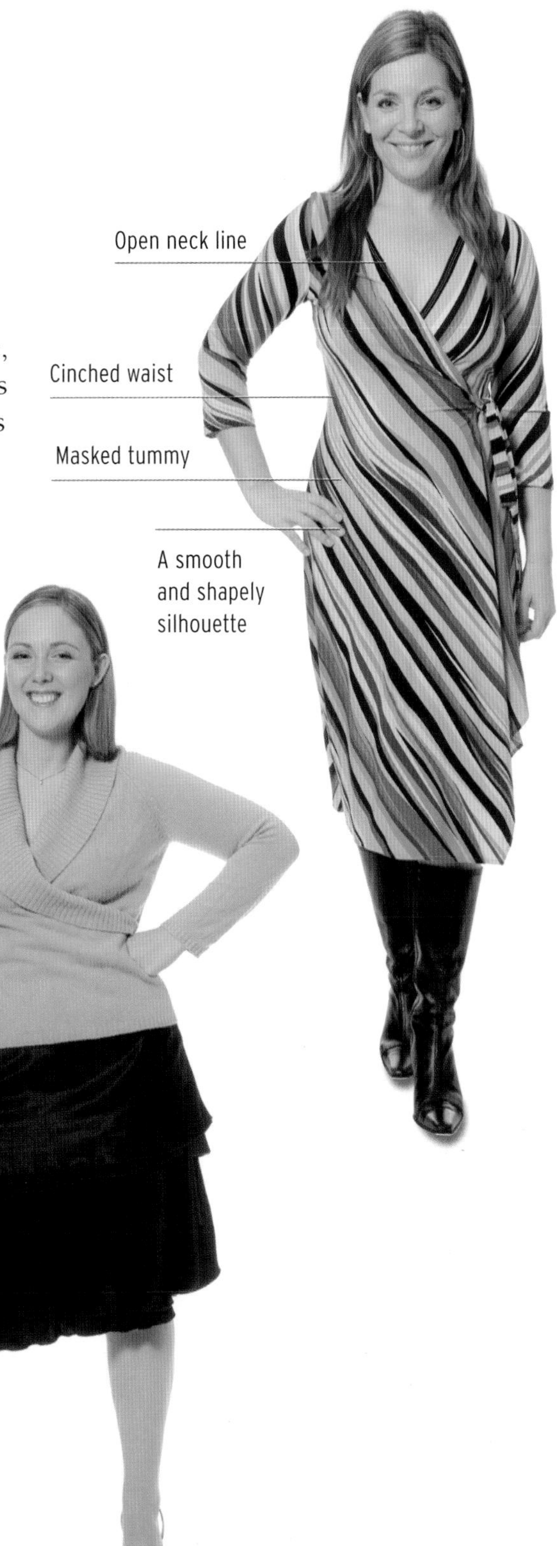

karen now

Here Karen shows us a faux wrap sweater that gives her some nice shape through the torso. Concerned to mask a more boxy top half, Karen here gets the **BENEFIT** of the wrap's **ACCENTUATION OF THE BUST** and empire waist. Its finer-gauge wool doesn't bulk her up but rather creates a **MORE REFINED SWEATER LOOK**, which she **POLISHES** even further with a brown silk tiered skirt. The skirt's tiers begin just after the widest part of her hip, effectively masking her hips and thighs (another problem area for Karen).

deborah now

Deborah, who can stand to add a little fullness to her slight figure, uses the **EMPIRE WAIST** to a different effect. Here, she dons a dress that poofs a bit below the cinch of the waist, **FLOWING** more fully about her torso and hips (great for pregnant ladies as well!). Its **FORMFITTING SHAPE** above the empire waist and her **REFINED** shoe choice keep its fullness looking less overwhelming on her frame, so she gets the most benefit from the dress's fuller design.

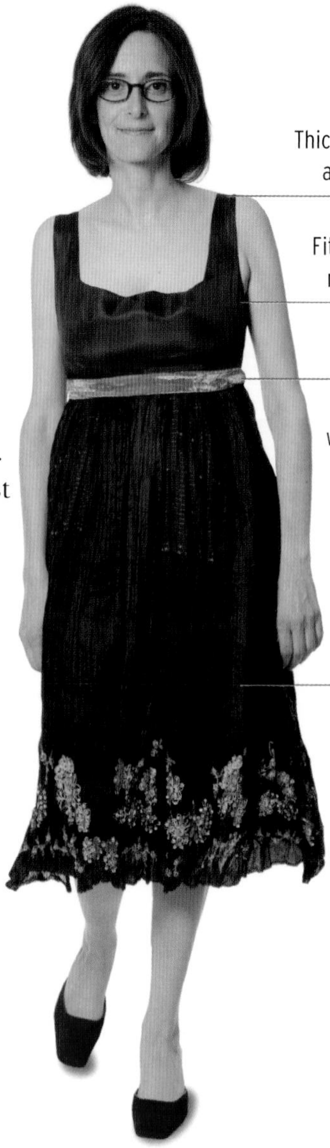

Thicker strap make her arms look less bony

Fit of the dress gives nice bust definition

Wide waistband works to define her waist so she is not overwhelmed by fabric

Fuller drape of this empire waist gives more substance to Deborah's frame

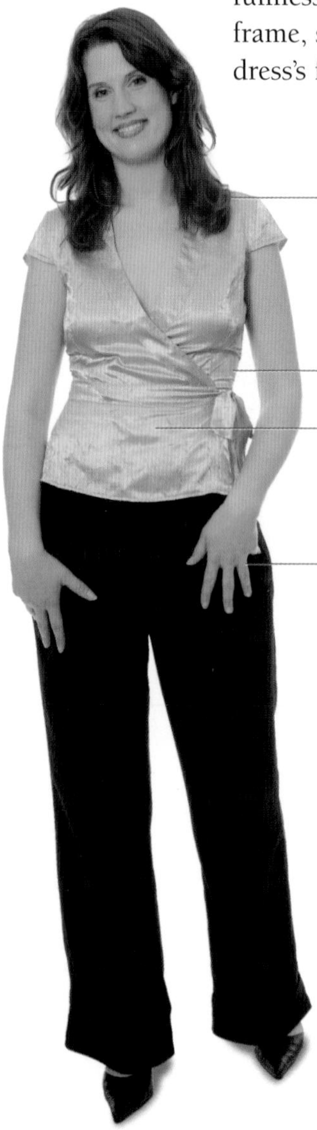

Open neck

Cinched waist

Smooth tummy

Easy flow over hips

morgan now

Lastly, here is Morgan in a **GREAT WRAP TOP** that draws our eye to her great **DÉCOLLETAGE** as it cinches her **NARROW EMPIRE WAIST** and flows smoothly over her tummy. **WHAT MORE COULD YOU ASK FOR** in any top?

The Last Word

Do you think you have the drift now? Wraps and empire-waisted tops provide some great figure fixes for all of us; try them on and see which ones work for you!

Things to look out for? Watch where a wrap top hits your torso. Not all wraps hit at the empire waist, and depending on your torso troubles, you don't want to get cut in the wrong place! The empire wrap is the most flattering for all, so aim for that.

Also, watch out for the pregnancy look. A stiffer fabric is often more likely to give you a nice A-line flare below the empire waist rather than a poofy look that might actually emphasize the fact that you are trying to hide something. (Though this style works great for pregnant women who want to accentuate their bellies!) Also, a wrap or other top that uses shirring across the tummy is a great way to wear sleeker cuts without having to expose too many rolls in the process. Shirring is a great friend, so use it liberally to camouflage your tummy.

In the next chapter, we'll talk about jackets, one of my favorite subjects. You'll discover how these versatile garments help us combat our arm and shoulder challenges, as well as take on boob and tummy troubles, all at the same time!

ULTIMATE TOP STYLE

Here are a few dos and don'ts to bear in mind when shopping for tops.

1. The good: Wrap tops, empire waists, shirring, formfitting sweaters, and layering can all work for you, enhancing your décolletage and disguising a problem belly and hips.
2. The bad: Bulky sweaters; boring, monochromatic, shapeless sweater sets; and poofier fits can make you look bigger than you are, and worse, frumpier than you'd ever want to be.
3. The ugly: Your sweaters should be as purposeful and constructive a part of your outfits as any other piece, not a utilitarian answer to being chilly. Saggy, drab cardigans, be gone!

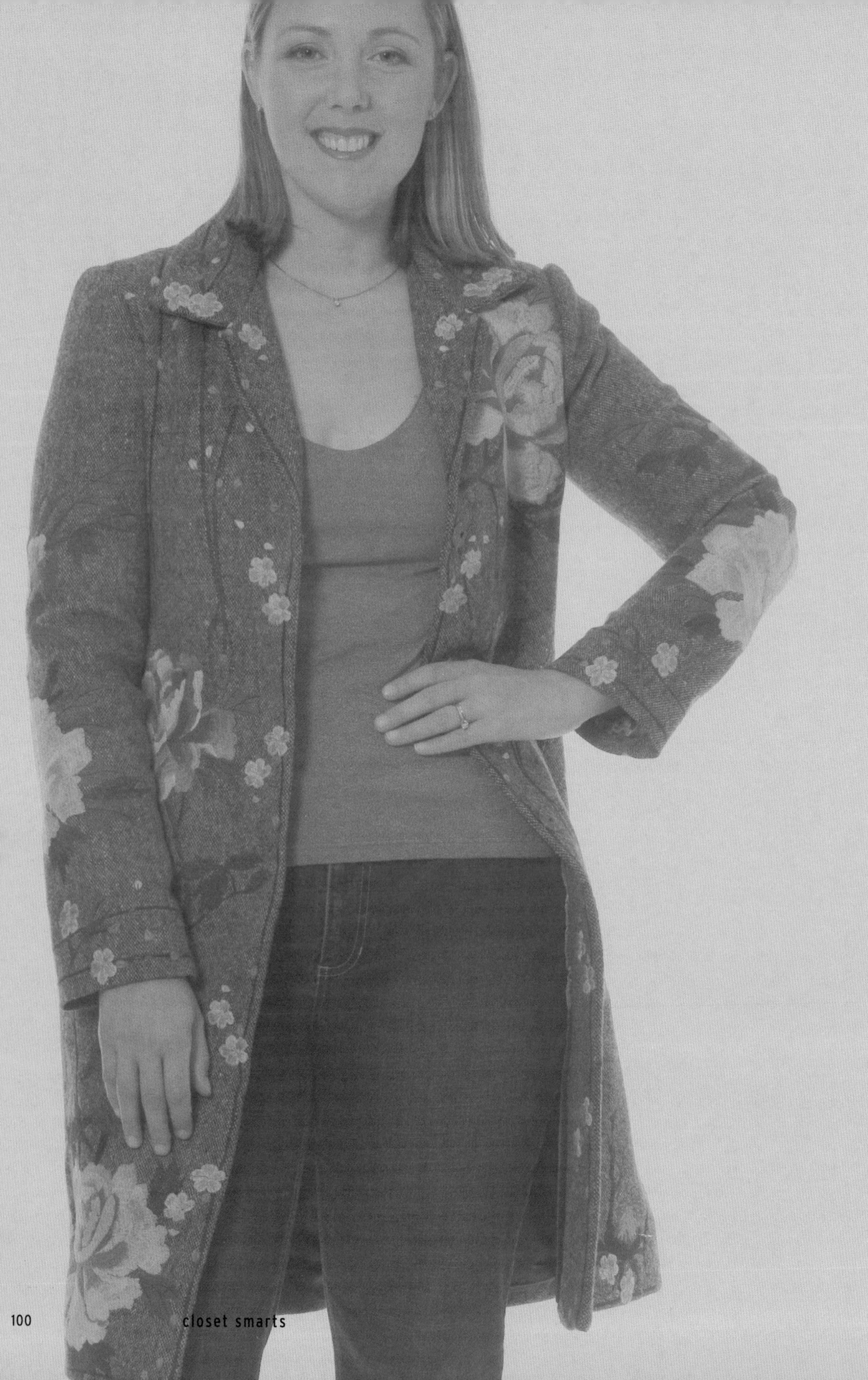

CHAPTER SIX

jackets:

They're Not Just for Cover Any More

6

This is the last chapter where we'll talk about our upper halves. Then it's time to take on the nether regions—our butts, thighs, and other choice phobic obsessions. Here we get to that final frontier of layer dressing for the top with a favorite item of mine—the jacket. Jackets deal with arm and shoulder issues, as well as boob and tummy issues, all at once! So, don't be surprised if you start to hear some of my recurring mantras. After all, you'll be more likely to remember these valuable tips and tricks when you are sorting through your closet, or out there shopping for the perfect jacket for you (which I hope you will be soon!). Jackets are my personal favorite because they can be so versatile, and they truly work with every shape. So let's see what a good jacket can do for *your* shape.

The Straight Jacket Fits! (Or Maybe the Cropped Look Is Better?)

You don't have to spend too much time with me before you get the idea that jackets are one of my number one fashion favorites. These are not the suity jackets of mid-thigh length, velvet lapels, and shoulder pads. You know, the ones that probably a good three-quarters of you still have at least one of hanging in your closet somewhere. Do yourself a favor right now, while I am with you. Put this book down for a minute (I know it's a page-turner), go over to your closet (stand up, I'm serious, right now), take these dinosaurs out of there, and simply throw them in the garbage!

No, they are never coming back into style. *No*, they are not solving your weak shoulder problem. And *no*, they don't make you look slimmer or taller by covering your butt and much of the top three-fourths of your body with a giant rectangle. And I don't care if it was really expensive (in the mid-80s). The look is over, and if it ever comes back, I will take personal responsibility for your losses.

That said, the kinds of jackets I get *excited* about are the great variety of shapes and styles that incorporate enough design details to totally assist in the revamping of your top half. There are truly enough styles and shapes of jacket out there to do the work of ten surgeons (which is never a good solution if you ask me—too expensive and too dangerous). As always, however, just to say it one more time, there are good jackets and bad jackets. The suity jackets I described earlier happen to be bad for everyone. But, even in the current world of fashion, a jacket that works wonderfully on one of us, may not suit another of us well at all.

CLOSET SMARTS STYLE: JACKET GEOMETRY

What is my basic approach in picking a jacket to suit a particular figure? The look I try to achieve with everyone I work with is that of two triangles whose tips meet at your waist, where the widest parts equal your shoulders and your hips and the narrowest part equals your waist. That is roughly the silhouette goal I am trying to achieve for each and every one of you.

Obviously, considering how many different kinds of you there are out there, not all of these triangles are going to be equilateral. There will be some isosceles amongst you, some right triangles, even a few scalenes. But you get the general picture—little in the middle, roughly proportionate on both ends, yes?

Find out how to use my Two-Triangle Theory to balance the proportions of your bottom half in chapter 7, beginning on page 127.

Since jackets are such a building block in suiting our top halves, we will spend some good pictorial time here instilling a little basic visual jacket-wearing wisdom. You'll see what kinds of jackets are likely to work for *your* figure, and which will truly undermine your aims at achieving a great look. So now to the pictorial segment of this program. Let's begin with Lily.

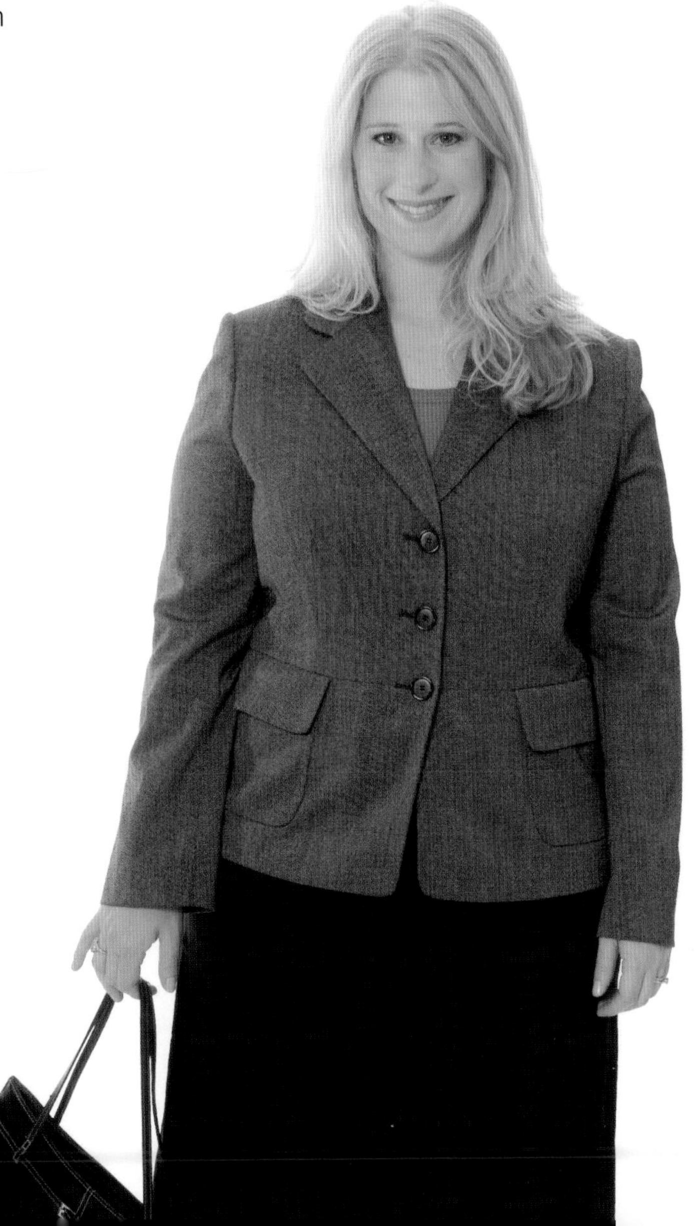

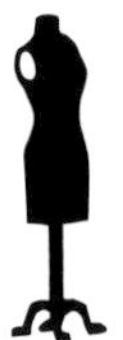

closet smarts: JACKETS FOR CURVES

THE CURVY GALS

Lily was sure an overly large black jacket was an indispensable part of her wardrobe. She could throw it over everything, and it literally covered everything—almost like a wet rag if you ask me.

lily before

As I've asked before in this fashion excursion, what is this jacket doing *for* Lily, besides simply *covering* her? Clothes should never just be tents for the body. Their utilitarian value can be far more complex than that. To break it down more specifically, this jacket is way too long on Lily. It hits her right at one of her widest parts: her hip and thigh area, drawing the eye *right* there. It overwhelms her top half in a giant shapeless rectangle, and, as we have seen, Lily has curves that can be put to good use. The shoulders on this monstrosity are way too large, setting Lily up for a further distortion of her proportion, making her look larger than she actually is. So again I ask, what is this jacket doing for her? Nothing, nada, zilch. Any chance that we have, we should be using clothes to help us *create* shape.

Let's take a look at some jacket looks that *do* work for Lily:

Shoulders that fit

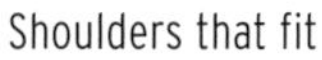

Open neckline draws attention to décolletage

lily now

Ahhh, now this cropped cotton twill number with a **LITTLE STRETCH** really works with Lily's figure, **ACCENTING THE GOOD PARTS** and downplaying the sketchier parts with the right fabric and design. To begin with, the jacket is cropped, hitting Lily at the narrowest part of her hips, the top. It is cinched at the waistline, drawing the eye toward the narrowest part of her torso (the empire waist), while allowing some room for her bust without squeezing and flattening her chest into a uniboob. The lower stance (where the top button of a jacket hits) and V-neck also work to open up and draw the eye to Lily's face and **DÉCOLLETAGE**, which is **ACCENTUATED** here by a V-neck Johnny collar top layered underneath. The overall look is **FITTED AND SHAPELY**, while providing the same kind of coverage (of tummy, arms, and bust) that Lily was trying to address with that first David Byrne number.

Clothes should never just be tents for the body.

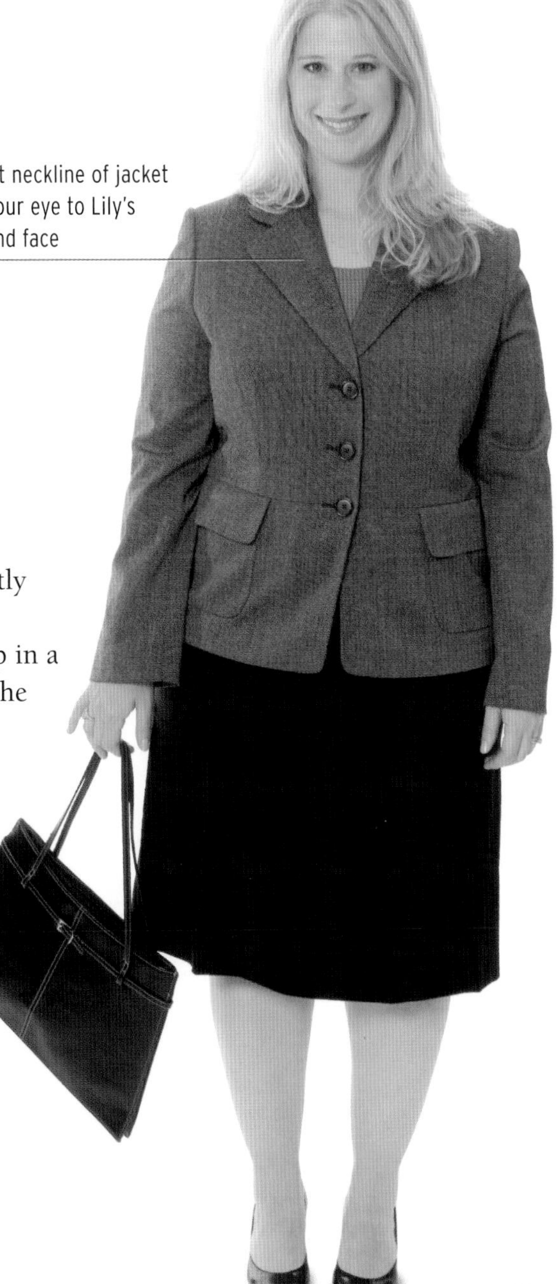

Low-cut neckline of jacket draws our eye to Lily's neck and face

lily now

Here Lily is again in a more suity number. This jacket is slightly boxier, but for the larger-breasted among us, a boxier fit can actually work to de-emphasize the chest, while hitting our hip in a **MORE FLATTERING PLACE** (skimming over the top here). Again, the stance of the jacket is low enough to open up Lily's décolletage, **DRAWING THE EYE** toward her face and neck, while darts throughout the jacket's torso provide a **GOOD WAIST SHAPE** in silhouette. This counteracts the boxiness of the jacket for the overall look. Done in a nice neutral gray, but accented by a fine-gauge, **SLIM-FITTING** cinnamon-pink sweater beneath and a very slimming pencil skirt in black, Lily's overall suity look is **QUITE SHAPELY**, while still providing the coverage she wants.

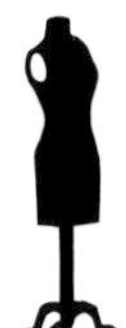

closet smarts:
JACKETS FOR CURVES

Yvette was not a big jacket fan when I met her, as she tended to think dressing in layers always had the effect of adding girth. (You can be quite assured that she now works the layering look to good advantage.) If anything, a jacket in Yvette's wardrobe was used as a decorative cover, like this fringed suede number.

Jacket cuts at Yvette's widest part

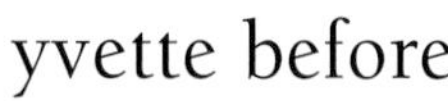

yvette before
This fringed suede number is one of Yvette's "cover-up" jackets.

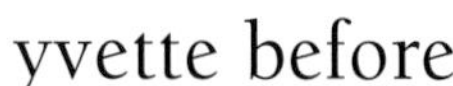

yvette before
This lightweight cotton jacket is another bad example. The more casual jacket is worn as a sort of cardigan over Yvette's dress, once more covering her up.

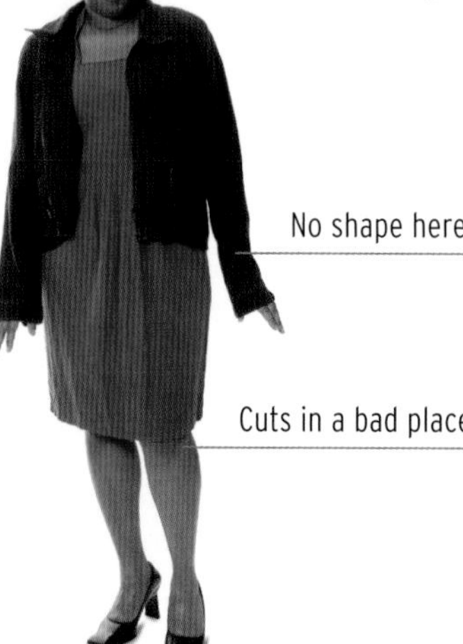

No shape here

Cuts in a bad place

Neither one is doing Yvette any favors. The suede fringed jacket acts more as an oversized shirt where the fringe, rather than adding an element of interest, really only seems to add the visual girth Yvette was concerned to avoid at the start. Indeed, the fringe seems to be the only design detail this jacket has to offer, as it is largely shapeless and boxy in the worst way. Yvette's boobs actually look larger here, while the cut of the sleeves leaves us with the impression that her arms are rather heavy as well.

The shorter cropped cotton jacket, while certainly boasting a more open neckline, also lacks shape and structure, the two most important things a jacket can add to our silhouettes. So what might be a workable alternative for Yvette? On the next two pages you'll see some great jacket looks for her.

Boxy jackets work for large-breasted women by allowing plenty of room for their boobs while not totally overwhelming their curves!

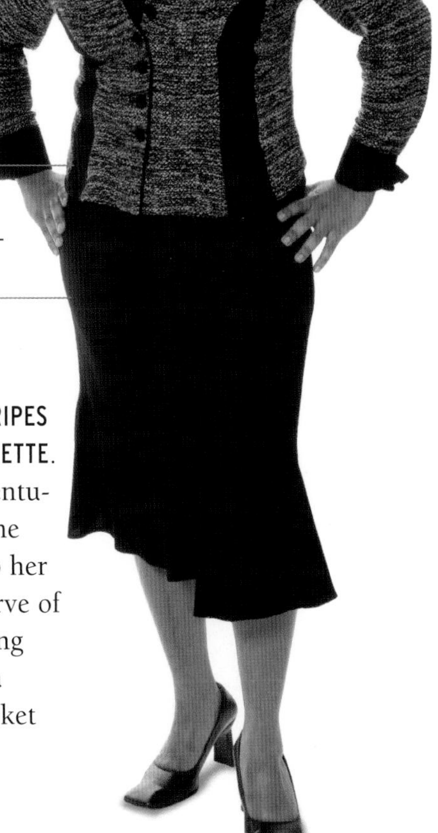

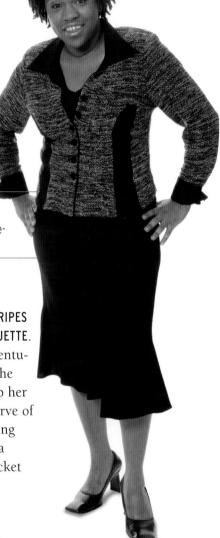

Vertical lines elongate the torso

Lycra adds good curve-hugging stretch

yvette now

This shapely bouclé salt-and-pepper jacket with **LYCRA AND RACING STRIPES** down the side has **ALL THE RIGHT MOVES** for Yvette's more **CURVY SILHOUETTE**. The fabric has the right combination of substance and stretch to accentuate, while reining in and smoothing Yvette's curves. Cinched below the bust, with a low stance to reveal **A BIT OF CLEAVAGE** and really open up her neck and chest, we are drawn into the outfit via Yvette's face. The curve of her bust is **HIGHLIGHTED** without being overly suggestive, and the racing stripes really help to show that she indeed *has* a waist—rather than a rectangle as a torso—without revealing any lumps or bumps. The jacket flows smoothly into a longer fluted skirt, with proportions that even out the width of her shoulder, hip, and knee, allowing for the curve of her hips without over-emphasizing them. We see **SKIN IN ALL THE BEST PLACES** (neck and chest, wrist, calf, and ankle), and Yvette looks **EFFORTLESSLY FABULOUS**.

yvette now

This more traditional suit is another good look for Yvette. It's paired with a shirred V-neck red mesh top beneath that shows some good curve through the bust but keeps coverage tasteful. Yvette gets a dash of hot color, even as she goes with the darker black power suit. The stance on this suit jacket is nice and low to show more of her layering choice and keep her top half open. It hits just at the top of her hip, and, combined with a straight-leg pant that falls from the widest part of her hip, her overall silhouette is **SMOOTH, CHIC, AND SLIMMING**. The shirring on the top really helps keep Yvette's tummy masked so she can wear her suit jacket open and feel **LESS BUTTONED UP** (not a favorite fashion choice for her).

Waist is created by darts

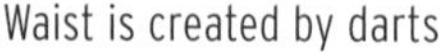

yvette now

Another **LOOK THAT WORKS** for Yvette is one I put together for her in chapter 3 when we talked about shoulders. This is a simple concept for her: a V-neck top that keeps her neck open, higher-stanced jacket that keeps her boobs in check while allowing some room for them (with darts and a good V-cut as well), **CINCHED WAIST**, and a jacket length that hits right at the top of her hips and is **COMPLEMENTED** by straight-legged pants that smooth the line of the hip and have an **OVERALL SLIMMING EFFECT**. As Yvette's image says in this photo, whala! How could it be so easy to take off ten pounds?!

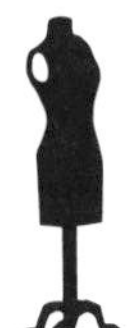

closet smarts: JACKETS FOR PROPORTION

PROPORTIONING TOPS AND BOTTOMS

Moving away from the bustier amongst us, let's take a look at Karen and Beth. Karen feels her shoulders are on the broader, slopier side, and that she needs to add structure to her upper half to keep it in proportion with the rest of her. Beth has a petite top and wider bottom, so she also struggles with proportion. Both look great in some of the jackets I put them in.

In Beth's case, our most important challenge will be evening out the width of shoulder versus hip. This can be achieved through a number of different jacketing strategies. We'll start with a skirted look. This is very similar to what I did with Yvette and the fluted skirt bottom. For those of us with larger hips, the flute at the bottom of even a curve-hugging skirt can really help proportion out hips and shoulders. Take this look for example.

Good structure in shoulder adds to overall proportion

Fluted bottom evens out proportion of larger hips

beth now

We use a **CROPPED JACKET** length here for Beth, and we *can* because of the higher rise of the skirt and its **CURVE-HUGGING** and fluted design details. Beth's petite top really calls for a smaller jacket. (Traditional-sized jackets really overwhelm her frame.) The cropped jacket has a better chance of fitting Beth's upper half, and it also avoids cutting Beth at her widest part (hips). So if we're going for fitted on the top (which we are), we have to be prepared to create **PROPORTION** on the bottom. Since the jacket cinches her **SMALL WAIST**, we have the perfect opportunity to allow some hip curve to show as part of building an overall **HOURGLASS** silhouette, and we can use the skirt's flute here to counterbalance too much hippiness. The jacket has some nice **STRUCTURED SHOULDERS** to build up Beth's frame and, as I always prefer, **A GREAT V-NECK** to keep the focal point at Beth's face and neck.

Another skirt and jacket option for Beth in the game of proportion, particularly where Beth's hips are concerned, is to use a fuller skirt combined with an even more fitted jacket (to counteract the overall impression of Beth being overwhelmed by too much fabric). Take a look.

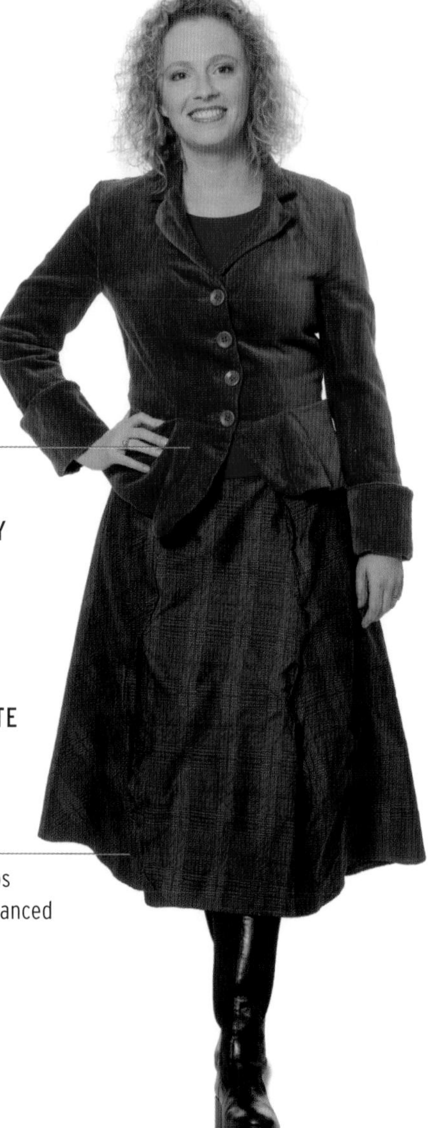

Asymmetrical jacket hem keeps eye moving rather than focusing on hips

beth now

In this ensemble, we pair an asymmetrical and **HIGHLY STRUCTURED** miniaturized **VELVET JACKET** with a fuller skirt (but with a lighter-weight material). The skirt's shape hides Beth's hips, while the jacket reminds us that she is indeed petite. Since the shoulders on the jacket are so pronounced, we get a nice **PROPORTIONATE LOOK** from head to toe, even with the width of the skirt's hem at a **FLARED** A-line.

Full skirt hides hips and is counter-balanced by fitted jacket

A jacket is a girl's best friend.

When it comes to pants and jackets, Beth has a few options as well. Here are two ways she can go.

beth now

In this outfit, we use a jacket whose single-button closure lands right at the empire waist, cinching Beth at her **NARROWEST** part and flaring out and over her hips. In this cut, **THE EYE IS DRAWN** to the low stance at the narrow empire waist. When we pair the jacket with straight-leg pants that also skirt over Beth's hip (i.e., *not accentuating it*), whala: Who said anything about big hips? Using the brown velvet with a **SOFT** (V-neck!) pink top beneath, echoed in the velvet pink shoe, we get an overall look of soft **FEMININE CURVES** that are perfectly in proportion and **TOTALLY FLATTERING** on Beth.

Another option for Beth is a slightly longer jacket that covers the hip, paired, again, with nice straight-leg pants that de-emphasize that extra curve of her hip.

beth now

In this outfit, we use a **LEATHER BLAZER** whose stiffness adds the **STRUCTURE** Beth needs on her top half, but whose cut is defined enough not to overwhelm her frame. (Think of Lily's big David Byrne jacket; this is not that!) In this case, the stance of the jacket is higher, **DRAWING THE EYE** to Beth's bust (accentuated, of course, by another V-neck that reiterates the jacket's cut). We leave it **OPEN** to show off the nice shirred-waist red top (the same as Yvette's, and doing wonders for masking that tummy). Paired with some **REFINED** black heels, the outfit looks **CHIC AS ALL GET OUT**, and once again, Beth looks **VERY WELL PROPORTIONED** in her overall silhouette. Ah, the wonders of proportion!

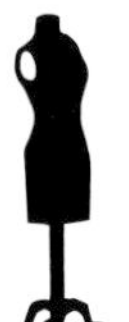

closet smarts: JACKETS FOR PROPORTION

As for Karen, who felt her biggest top-half problem was being too broad and rounded, we can use a jacket to add some more structure and shape. Since Karen is also concerned with the thickness of her thigh area, we want to be sure that we combine our top and bottom efforts to make an overall proportioned silhouette and keep the top half speaking with the bottom half. Karen's original idea about jackets was that any jacket might add the extra coverage she wanted on the top. But take a look at the contours of *this* jacket.

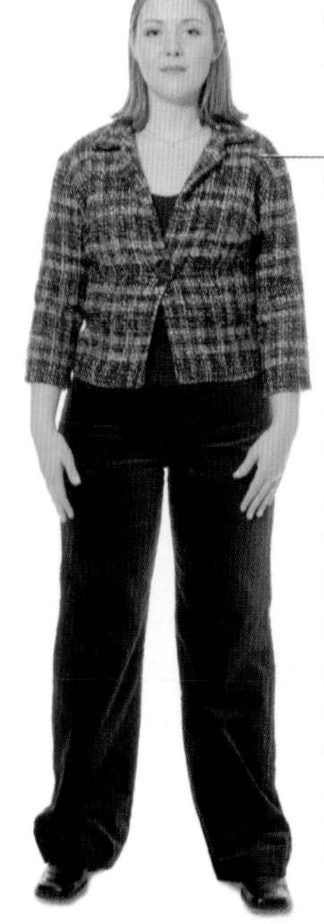

Ill-fitted shoulder seams emphasize round appearance of arms

karen before

As we saw in the shoulders chapter, the lines of this jacket do nothing for Karen's concern about a rounded/broad or sloping silhouette. Since its shoulder line is so far *off* the square of her shoulder, the jacket actually makes Karen look *more* broad-shouldered than she is. The cropped shape can indeed work for her, but certainly not with pants that accentuate her hips and thighs, as these do.

karen now

A **BETTER LOOK** overall for Karen can be found in the jacket we saw on Beth on page 111. Here, the cinch of the jacket is at the empire waist (the narrowest part), we have a **HIGHLY STRUCTURED** shoulder, and the **CROPPED SHAPE** cascades over the hips. Combined with an A-line skirt, we remold Karen's shape into something **PLEASING TO THE EYE,** covering all the trouble spots (shoulders, hips, and thighs) and creating a **GREAT PROPORTION** between shoulder, waistline, and knee.

Full skirt hides hips and is counter-balanced by fitted jacket

karen now

For a more everyday skirted look, we try a similar silhouette with an A-line skirt and boots and whala! **ANOTHER WINNING COMBO** for fighting Karen's figure phobias.

Figure-structuring jacket adds a waist, square shoulders, and skims over tops of hips

A-line skirt masks hips

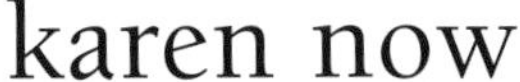

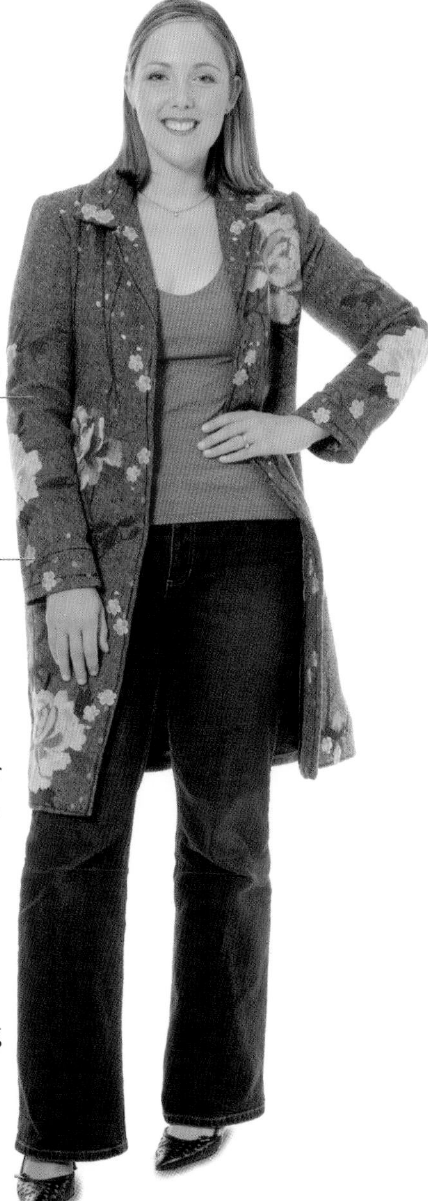

Combined with a figure-hugging top the jacket does not overwhelm her

A larger jacket with fit and style can be used to hide hip area

karen now

Karen can also use a longer jacket to address her concerns about shoulders and thigh width. Here we see her in a **FIGURE-HUGGING** pink scoopneck that shows off her great **FLAT TUMMY**. The scoop keeps her **DÉCOLLETAGE** open (and not lost in the cover of the longer jacket). Combined with straight-legged dark denim jeans that smooth out and elongate her thighs while nicely skirting over the hips and a refined pair of black heels, Karen looks **PUT TOGETHER, CHIC**, and ever so **WELL PROPORTIONED**.

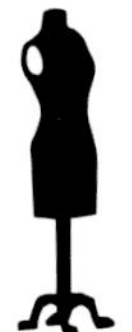

closet smarts:
JACKETS FOR PROPORTION

HOW TO KEEP AN HOURGLASS HALF FULL

For Amy, who has been blessed with a well-proportioned silhouette from the outset in the form of an hourglass figure, the trick will be making sure the jacket she chooses makes the most of that shape. We don't want to see it overwhelmed. Rather, we want to see it *accentuated* and as always, *enhanced*, because that's the work that clothes should be doing! For comparison's sake, I have two black jacketed looks to show you—the wrong one, and the right one. Let's start with this number, pulled out of her closet, dating back to the early '90s. Not the *worst* era in jacket dressing, but clearly not quite fully devoid of its '80s forebears.

Jackets should accentuate, not overwhelm.

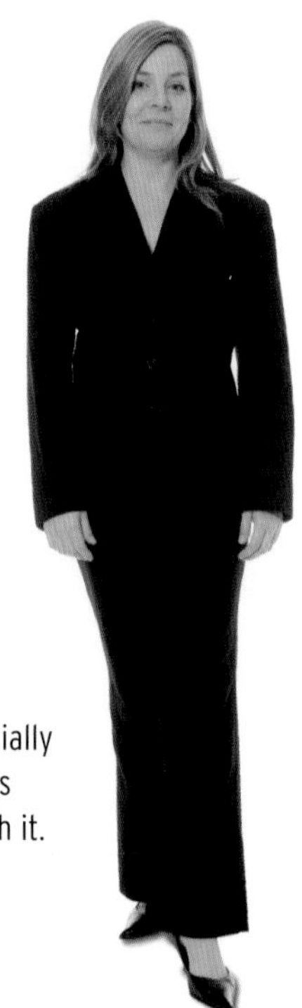

amy before

The jacket shape on Amy in this photo is very long and straight through the torso, with shoulder pads included, and it's largely shapeless through the bodice. Though there are some darts at the front waist, they are low, having the effect of over elongating the waist. There are no darts about the bust, so, combined with the shoulder pads, the amount of fabric at the top of Amy's torso is overwhelming on her frame, especially in basic black, and it certainly does nothing to show her shape beneath it.

Now let's move to current times. In the next shot, Amy models another basic black jacket, but just look at the difference.

amy now

You get the impression that Amy is wearing this jacket, rather than vice-versa. This one has no built-in shoulder pads (though certainly some **STRUCTURE** through the shoulders), a higher stance and shorter placket, darts at the bust, and a more **CINCHED WAISTLINE**. The styling at the bottom has almost a peplum type of cut that flows out over her hips, simultaneously creating and accentuating a nice waist and skimming over the hips (rather than cutting them awkwardly or simply covering over them and potentially bulking them up). Amy certainly looks suity **CHIC** with the bootleg pants to finish off the **HOURGLASS PROPORTIONS** and a refined black heel.

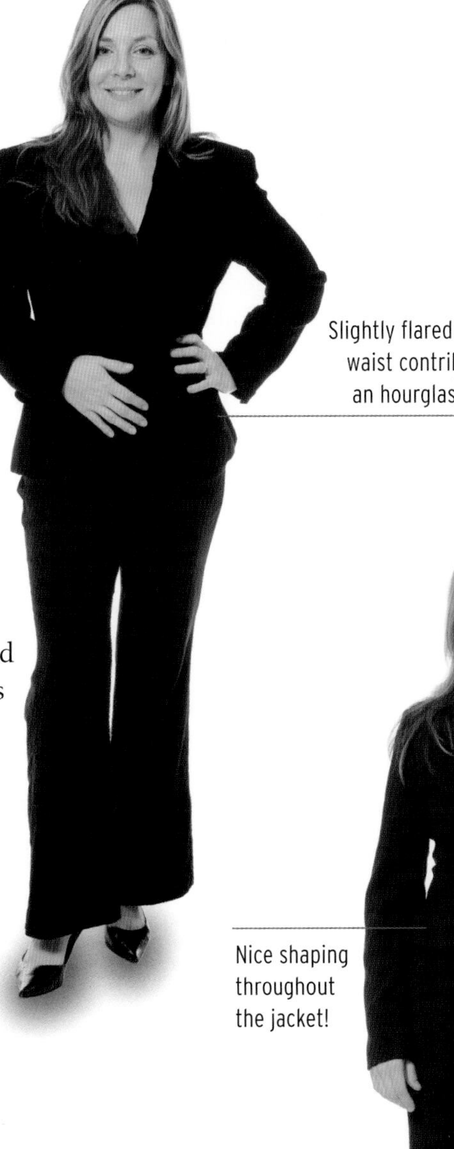

Slightly flared peplum waist contributes to an hourglass shape

Let's take one more look at Amy in work mode before we move on.

Nice shaping throughout the jacket!

amy now

Here's a great skirt-and-jacket work option for Amy. This cropped and cinched ensemble **HUGS EVERY INCH** of Amy's curves. The jacket's cropped length allows the skirt to do the work of elongating Amy's silhouette nicely and balancing out her hips with a slight flare at the bottom. From shoulder to hip to mid-calf, Amy is **PERFECTLY SUITED** here—not overwhelmed in fabric, but nicely covered and even sultry.

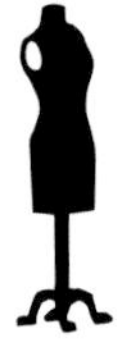

closet smarts:
JACKETS FOR BIG BOTTOMS

MAKING THE MOST OF TALL

What about one of our taller models, Morgan? Besides her height, which she is not overly troubled by, she considers her booty to be the hardest element to incorporate into her overall silhouette, so we'll want to keep this proportion issue in mind when looking for the right jacket look for her.

One option for this framework is the idea I used on Beth earlier—the fuller skirt, combined with a well-fitted and/or asymmetrical jacket to keep the eye interested, but not overly focused on the trouble spots. Because Morgan is taller than Beth, there is also less danger of her becoming overwhelmed in fabric if we use a fuller skirt, or a jacket with more design elements. Check out this suited look on Morgan.

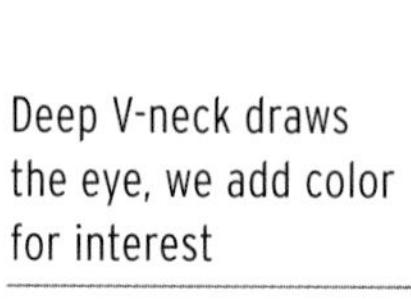
Deep V-neck draws the eye, we add color for interest
Scalloped hem smoothes over hips

morgan now

The **ASYMMETRICAL JACKET** does wonders to draw the eye to its cinch (through Morgan's **NARROW WAISTLINE**), while skirting over and beyond her wider parts. The skirt gets fuller as it travels down the leg for an **OVERALL SLIMMING LOOK** through the thigh and butt, though it certainly accommodates some girth there quite well. The glen plaid is busy and small enough to **MASK ANY PROBLEMS** as well, and we add a **STRIKING** turquoise top underneath for interest. A refined-toed shoe helps to clench the overall slimming look, and Morgan appears quite put together and **FIGURE-FLAWLESS** in the ensemble.

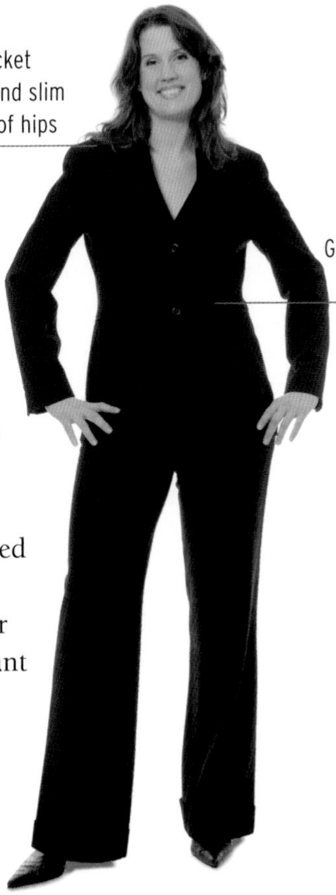

Longer flared jacket works to cover and slim the appearance of hips

Good shape through the waist

As for a more suity jacket look for Morgan, we tried this classic black suit jacket and pants on her for size.

morgan now

Again, we're focused on **ACCENTUATING** Morgan's best parts (long legs, nice waistline, and **WELL-PROPORTIONED** top) and masking her sensitive parts (butt/hips/thigh area). So the jacket we choose here has a high stance (drawing us to her neckline and face) and is well shaped throughout the torso, flaring slightly out and over the hips. Because of Morgan's height, she does well to wear a longer jacket, but again, not too long, as we don't want that jacket hitting at her widest part. Rather, we want to see a jacket **SKIMMING AND SHAPING** her midsection. This jacket falls perfectly over her hips, ending just where a pair of **NICELY MATCHED** straight-legged pants continue the smooth line straight down her long leg to a **LOVELY REFINED HEEL**, achieving the perfect pairing of coverage and enhancement. She looks **MARVELOUS**!

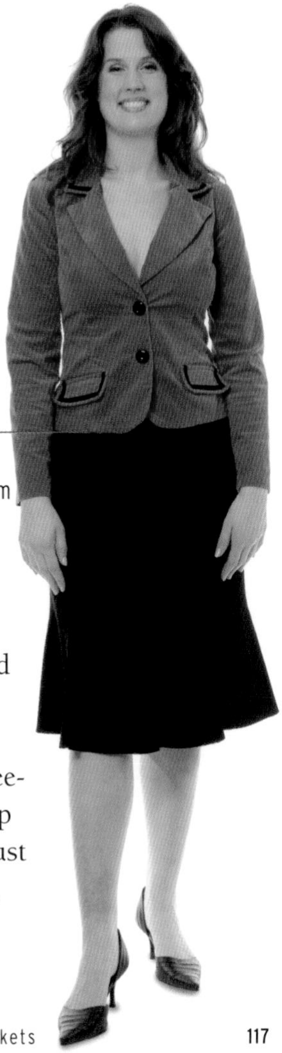

Cinched waist and cropped hem creates curves

morgan now

As for **MAKING THE MOST** of Morgan's curves, we also tried this cinched vintagey velvet jacket combined with a flute-bottomed skirt (a strategy we've tried on both Yvette and Beth as well). Here we actually allow for the **NATURAL CURVE** of the hip/butt area, but counter it with a very visually cinched waist and knee-length fluted skirt to fill out a well-proportioned look from top to bottom. After all, hips are **A THING OF BEAUTY**, it's all about just getting them to *fit in*. Morgan looks truly **FEMININE AND CURVY**, without being overly curvy (read heavy) in this ensemble.

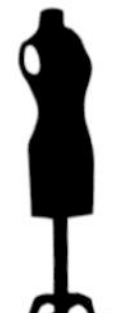

closet smarts:
JACKETS FOR BIG BOOBS

AND MAKING THE MOST OF SMALL

So how about our slimmer models, Deborah and Supriya, both of whom could definitely take advantage of a jacket's structure-providing and shape-enhancing qualities. Supriya has added concerns about being long-waisted and having larger breasts. As far as her bust is concerned, making sure she fits into tops without either being squished into a uniboob or having her bust overemphasized are the caveats that we'll keep in mind as we look for jackets. And we'll address Supriya's concern about long-waistedness through layering techniques as well as the length of jacket we choose for her silhouette.

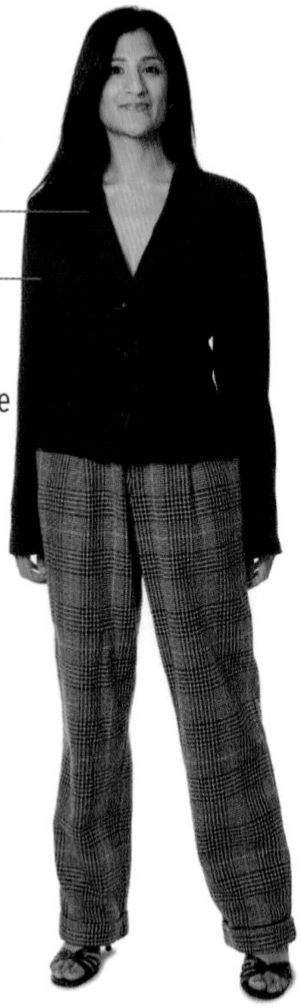

Stance is too low for her bust

Lighter fabric droops rather than adding structure and substance

supriya before

In this first shot, we've certainly done Supriya's figure no favors. The jacket's low stance, while seemingly providing more room for her boobs, tends to overwhelm them with too much fabric while simultaneously elongating her waist, just the opposite effect from what she would like to achieve. The lighter-weight fabric does nothing to enhance Supriya's figure, and despite its tailored cut, the jacket ends up just drooping on her, rather than adding any structure or shape.

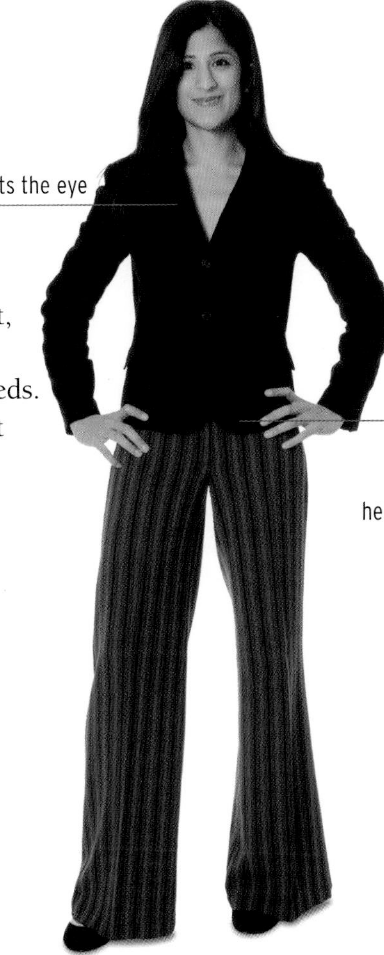
V-neck attracts the eye
Cropped fit shortens her long waist

supriya now

When we swap Supriya into this **FITTED** black velvet jacket, the effect is quite the opposite. The heavier fabric really provides the **STRUCTURE AND SHAPE** that Supriya's figure needs. With the higher stance, Supriya's boobs are contained, but not smooshed, and our eye is still drawn to the bust via a **NICE DEEP V-NECK**. The more cropped cut of the jacket combined with a pair of flat-front trousers shortens her waist's appearance, but makes the most of a **LONG-LEGGED SILHOUETTE** (especially with the wide pinstripe).

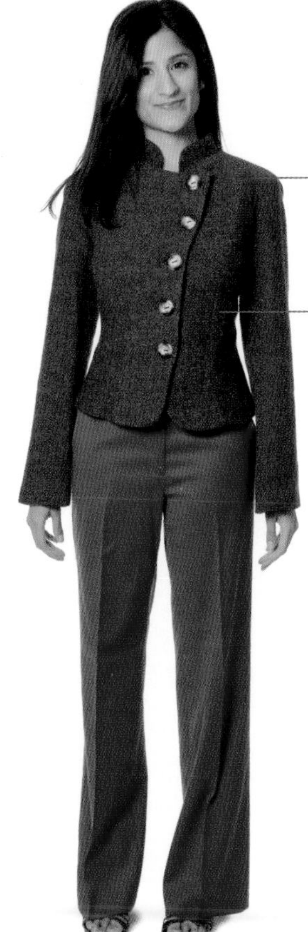
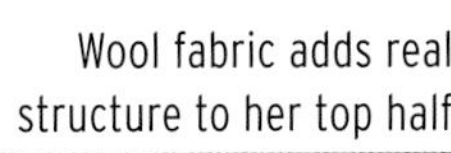
Wool fabric adds real structure to her top half
Shape-cinching waistline

supriya now

We also tried this Nehru-collared jacket on Supriya, which looked great. In this look, Supriya gets **GOOD COVERAGE** through her bust area, where the stiffer wool fabric contains her while maintaining (and adding) some **STRUCTURE** and shape. The jacket is **WELL TAILORED** through the waist, so she is not lost in the high-necked style, but she actually **BENEFITS** from its shoulder- and top-enhancing girth. The asymmetrical button placket also breaks up the potential line of a uniboob, and the **SCALLOPED HEM** artificially shortens the line of her waist. What a lot of work one little jacket can do!

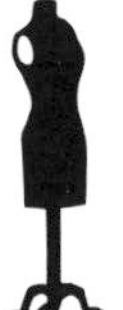

closet smarts:
JACKETS FOR SMALL BODIES

Deborah needs a jacket that fits her small frame, while perhaps adding some shape to her otherwise wispy silhouette. The suit she had in her closet, as you'll see in the next photo, seems to achieve exactly the opposite.

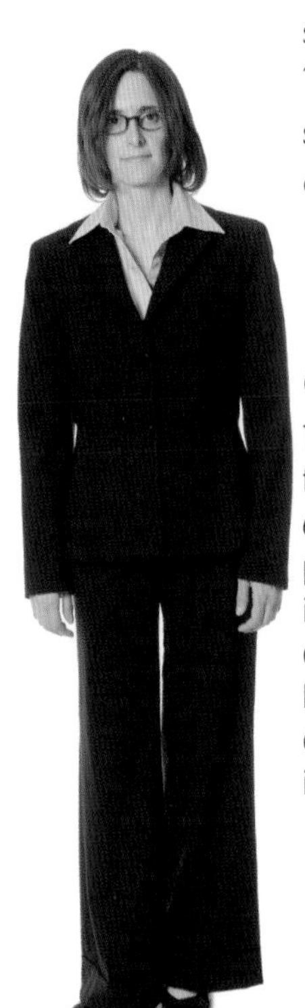

deborah before

Though certainly adding width to Deborah's frame, this oversized and overly long jacket is overly *everything* as far as I'm concerned. These shoulder pads *completely* overwhelm her proportions, the waist is far too low on her frame, elongating her torso disproportionately, and the length (to mid-thigh) also has the effect of overwhelming her frame rather than enhancing it. You really get the feeling that this suit is wearing her.

Low stance cinches her waist and raises it

Scalloped hem creates shape through her hips

deborah now

We got a **MUCH BETTER** result when we tried this miniaturized velvet number. Its single-button closure (with accompanying low stance), creates a good **WAIST** for Deborah. The effect is **ENHANCED** by its scallop-edged bottom, helping to create the appearance of some kind of hip—not to mention the great deep green color and the **HIGHLY ORIGINAL** embroidery as points of outfit interest. We layered the top here with a **FORMFITTING** brown camisole and velveteen **SLIM-FITTING** pants.

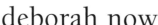

Jackets can add shape to a skinny silhouette.

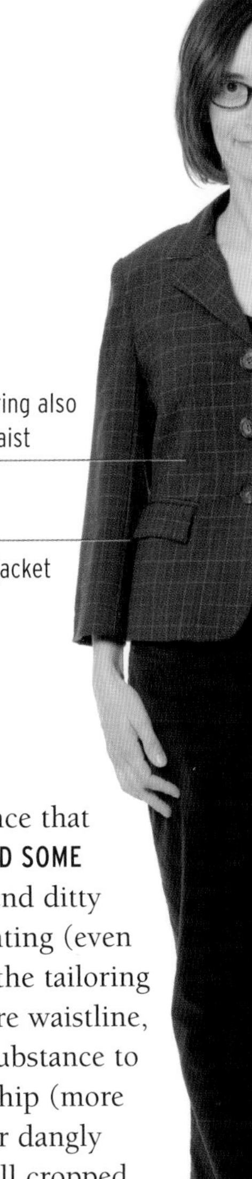

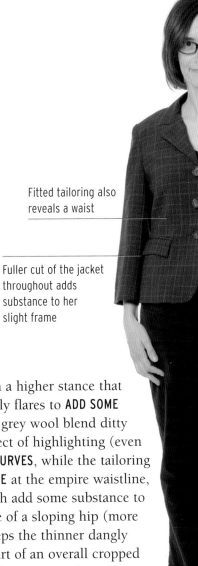

Fitted tailoring also reveals a waist

Fuller cut of the jacket throughout adds substance to her slight frame

deborah now

Another good jacket for Deborah is one with a higher stance that cinches closer to the empire waist and slightly flares to **ADD SOME STRUCTURE** to her torso. This light heathered grey wool blend ditty does the trick. The higher stance has the effect of highlighting (even while covering!) her bust by **SHOWING SOME CURVES**, while the tailoring of the jacket still creates a **CINCHED SILHOUETTE** at the empire waistline, and enough **FLARE** through the bodice to both add some substance to her wispy middle and to give the appearance of a sloping hip (more curve artifice). The shorter sleeve length keeps the thinner dangly appearance of Deborah's arms in check as part of an overall cropped and tailored look that really suits her slight frame. Again here, we use the stiffer velveteen pants to add some **SUBSTANCE AND STRUCTURE** to her legs' silhouette, and they look good combined with the jacket.

The Last Word

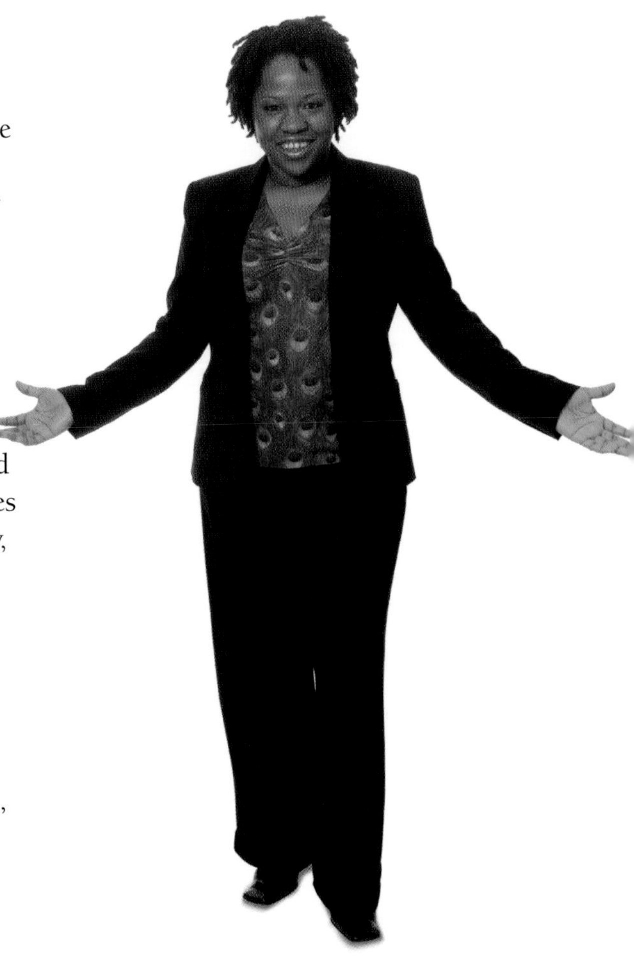

Now that we've taken quite an extensive tour along the great hall of jackets, I hope you will agree with me that they are one of the most versatile elements you can add to your wardrobe to get the most out of it. They truly are a woman's best friend, and their power to shape the silhouette *you* want to inhabit should not be underestimated.

Take some of the tips you've learned in these pages about which jacket shapes might enhance *your* figure type, and try, try, try on as many jackets as you can find at your local shopping haunts. You'll start to see the variety of looks you can pull off, and you'll learn just how central jacketing can be to pulling other elements of your wardrobe together. Whether you like pants, skirts, or dresses, a jacket can get you more outfits in combination than any other element in your wardrobe. Just make sure the jacket fits!

Just make sure the jacket fits!

This chapter concludes our section on the upper half. Now it's time to explore our Closet Smarts options for the *lower* half—butts, thighs, and legs. As with our tops, you'll find plenty of ways to create the silhouette you want with the figure you have—and a little style savvy. We'll take a look at the best strategies for smoothing out your hips, thinning your thighs, and enhancing your assets as you choose the right pants and skirts for your body type. So read on!

ULTIMATE JACKET STYLE

Make sure your jackets work for you by keeping these pointers in mind.

1. First and foremost, throw out those shoulder-padded, velvet-trimmed, mid-thigh-length '80s atrocities—*now*! The Goodwill is waiting!
2. Don't be afraid to try on lots and lots of jackets (keeping in mind the tips for those basic shapes that suit *your* shape, of course). Before you know it, your eyes will become trained to pick your workable styles off the rack on your first go-round.
3. Keep the length of the jacket in proportion to *your* length.
4. A deep V-neck is a great look to pair with a jacket because it keeps the neckline open and draws the eye to that lovely décolletage.
5. Fitted jackets and skirts that flute at the hem are a great way to smooth out and add proportion to a curvier shape or to *create* the perfectly proportioned hourglass you've always wanted!

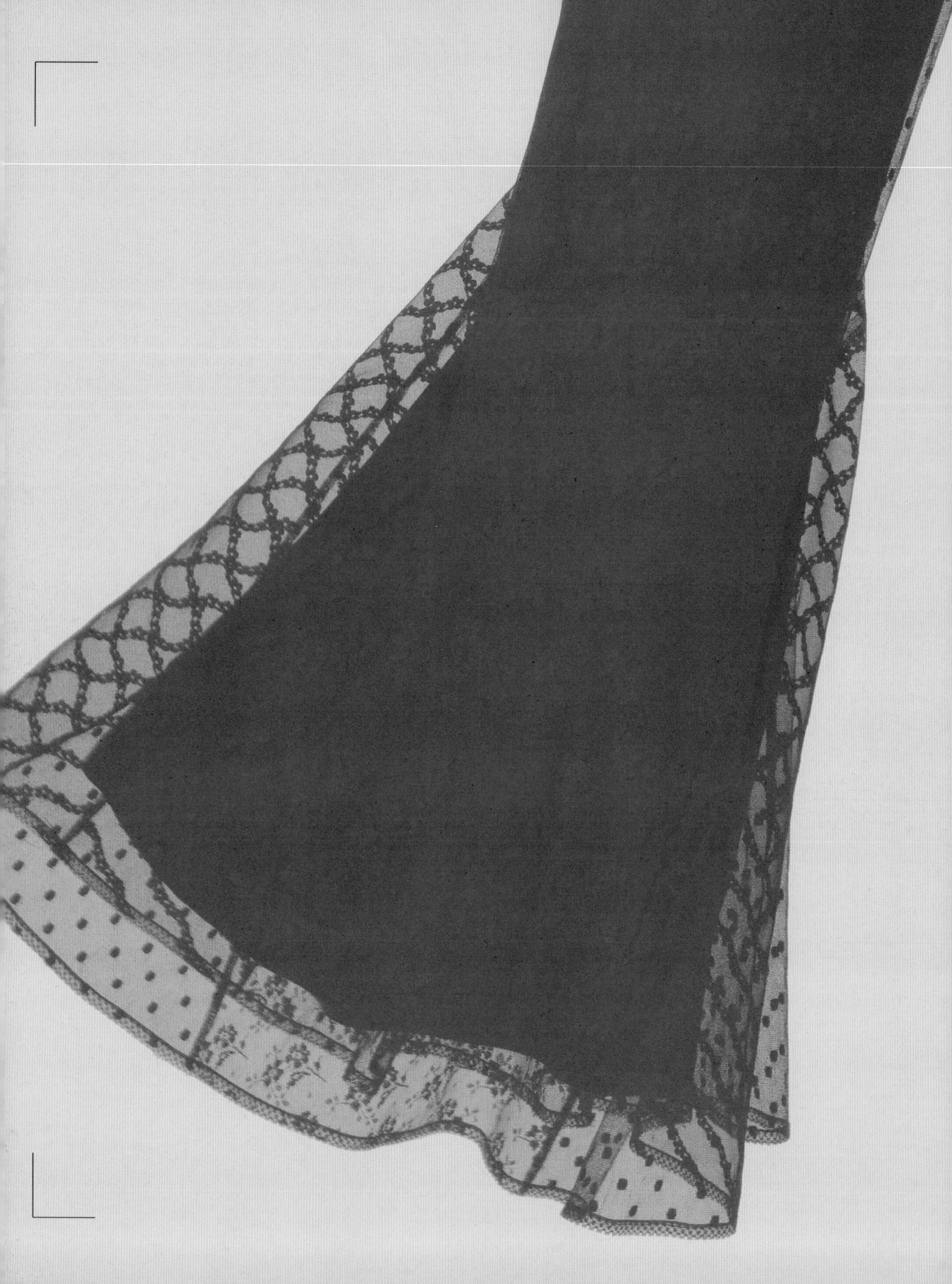

part two: THE LOWER HALF

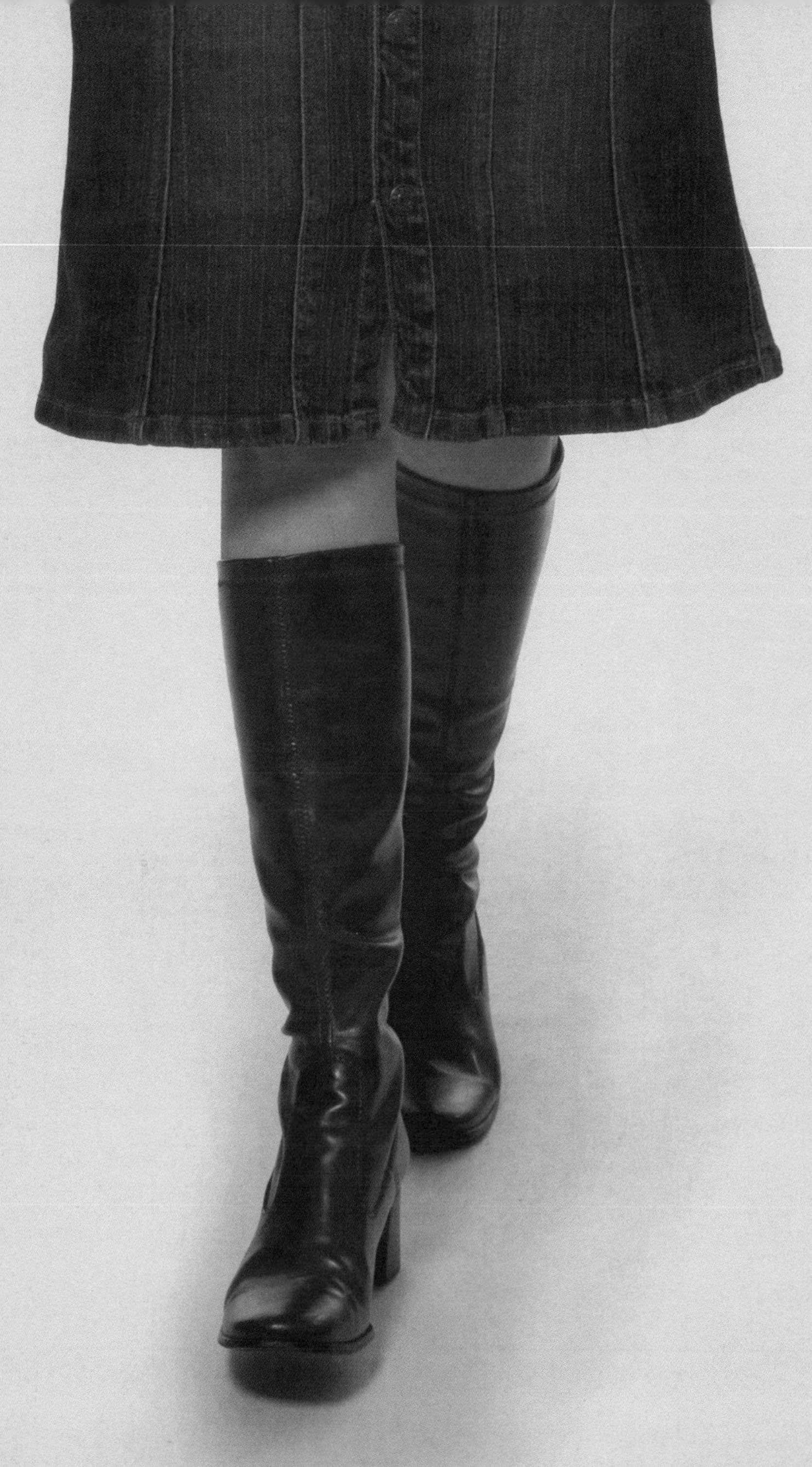

CHAPTER 7

7

the art of proportion

The Two-Triangle Theory

We must start this section of the book with a reminder about the most important thing for sculpting your most flattering silhouette—*proportion*. It is the mother of all fashion tips and tricks, and the moment you lose sight of it is the moment you will find yourself back in the '80s, shaped, most probably, like an ice cream cone—big shoulder pads, skinny tapered ankle pants—the disaster of all silhouettes.

As we take a closer look at the proportions of your nether regions, the areas to keep your eye on are your natural waist (where does it fall?), your hip size (especially in regard to your shoulder width), your thighs (how do they work with your hips?), and your knees, calves, and ankles (are they thick or thin, but more important, are they in proportion with the rest of your nether regions?). I'll show you how to look at all of these areas together as a single part, so you can really see your bottom half, maybe for the first time ever.

You see, though we are used to scrutinizing our bodies part by part, when you are dressing your body to disguise your less favorable parts, it's not always really necessary to worry about each part individually. It's the overall package that shows up on the radar, and that is why we are focusing on *silhouette* here. For example, you may think you have fat knees, but if they're actually in proportion with the size of your calves, from the outsider's perspective, we can make that part of your body work well in your overall appearance.

So sure, go on hating your knees if you like, but take heart from my promise that other people really aren't scrutinizing each and every individual part of you. They are taking you in *as a whole*, and if you are put together proportionately, their eyes are not drawn to look at those vulnerable parts, even if you're secretly burning up about them. Trust me on this. As I said at the beginning, I don't expect to talk you out of your body phobias; I have them, too. But I *do* expect to convince you that you can look great despite them!

I'm sure you remember how I insisted in Part One that people with heavier arms can wear short sleeves. (It's all about where the sleeve cuts on your arm and where the eye is drawn.) And I pointed out how a V-neck always draws the eye toward the universally good décolletage and the face, rather than to trouble spots. In this part of the book, I will have similar advice about your nether regions.

People really aren't scrutinizing each and every individual part of you.

A Woman's Curves Are a Thing of Beauty

The waist and the hips are a huge focus for the lower part of the body. They are the beginning of the bottom half, where it all begins, and as such, they are universally troublesome for most women, and especially for women who have generous hips. How did we get to think of these lovely curves as so problematic? I happen to think that a woman's curves are a thing of beauty. The only problem I can see with them is that they are often out of proportion with some of our other curves and squares. But we have clothing to help us out of this fix so let's use it to best effect!

Though you may think that the bottom half is much harder to address than the top half, there's a design trick that can help you. I believe it works for every woman, once it's properly adjusted for her particular issue or issues (long- or short-waisted, big- or small-hipped, thick- or thin-thighed). As I mentioned earlier, this theory of figure proportion is what I like to call the Two-Triangle Theory. It's the idea that, as we build our silhouettes using the clothing strategies I have outlined throughout this book, the goal is to construct a figure that roughly appears as two triangles meeting tip to tip in the middle (at your waist).

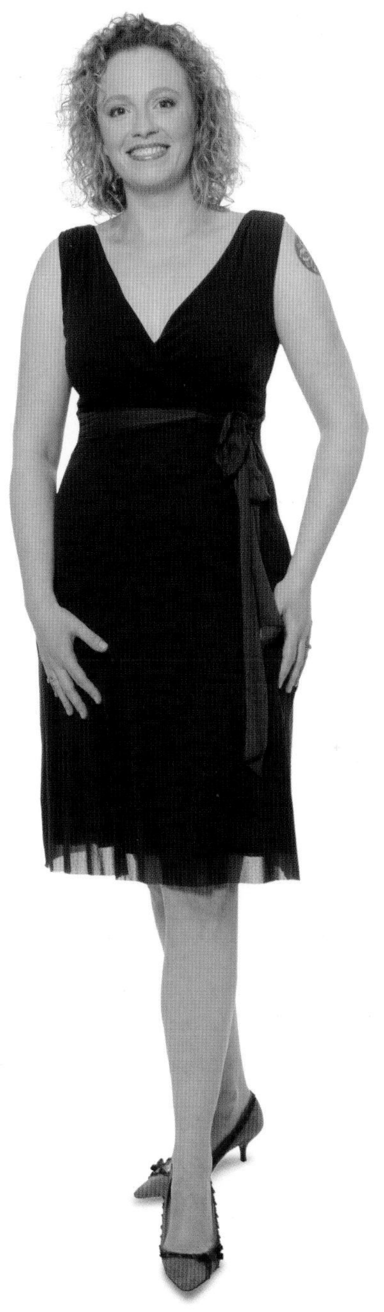

The Last Word

As long as you take this two-triangle image (below) into the dressing room (or your closet) with you, you will find it much easier to stay on the right track. So with that image in mind, let's revisit our models and their nether regions in the next two chapters.

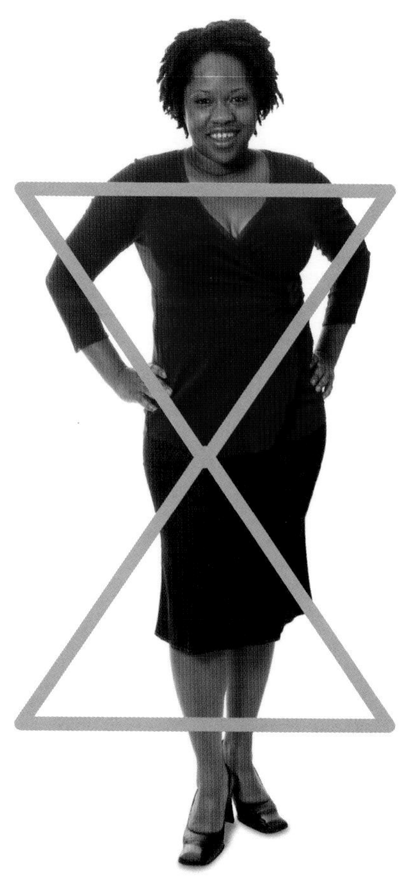

THE TWO-TRIANGLE THEORY.
Use this simple shape to create your perfect silhouette.

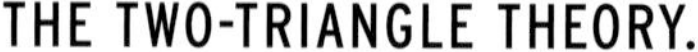

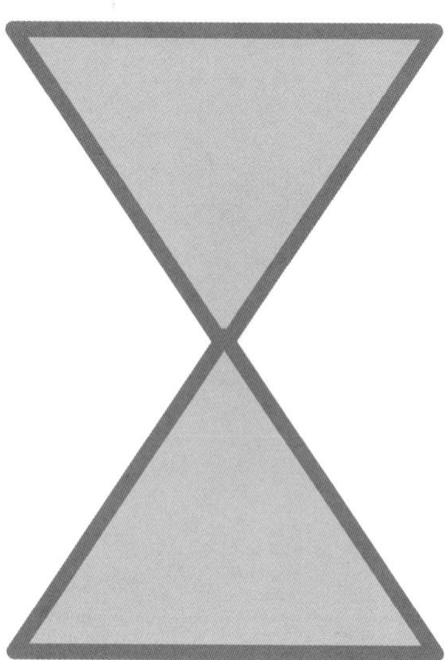

We've already talked a lot in the first part of the book about our models' various figure challenges and even some of the figure fixes that applied to more than their top halves (after all, waists and tummies are pretty closely related). Now we'll look at their particular fashion challenges as we take a look at good and bad pants options and good and bad skirt and dress looks. Once again, you'll be able to find your own figure challenges among our models and take the figure-fixing wisdom I'm about to show you along with you the next time you shop or get dressed.

ULTIMATE FIGURE FIXES

How do you use the Two-Triangle Theory? There are thee basic figure fixes you should bear in mind when you use your clothes to create a proportionate shape:

1. Create a waist (where you want it).
2. Mask large hips by using the breadth of your shoulders and the cut/flare of your pants or skirt to de-emphasize width in the middle of your figure.
3. Keep all parts of your silhouette proportionate within this larger outline. (The triangles should of course be equilateral.)

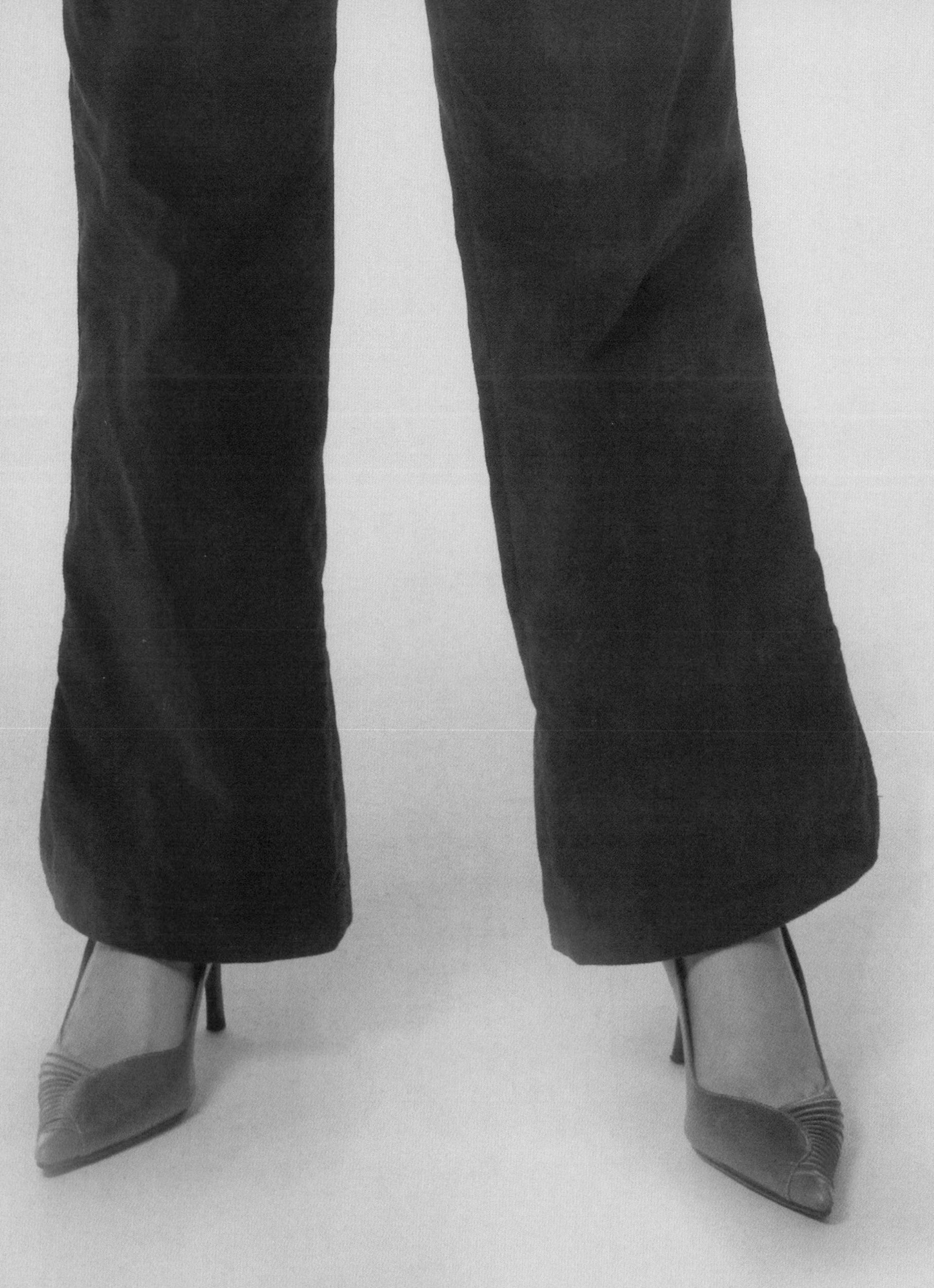

CHAPTER EIGHT

8

the pants dance:

Waisting Away and Other Critical Issues

In this chapter, we will explore all that can go right and wrong with pants as we struggle to find where a waistline should fall to best mask our tummies, how to fit our hips into the bigger picture, how to deal with thick thighs or disproportionate butts, and how to hide the lumps and bumps that tend to gravitate toward our lower halves over time. Oh yes, they are troublesome, but they are fixable flaws. And as always, it's all about proportion and silhouette.

CLOSET SMARTS STYLE

Counterintuitive as it may be—and I face this with all the women I work with in my business—showing *more* is actually the best way to make yourself appear smaller. All you really have to worry about is using your clothes to create the shape you want. Whether you're a size 16 or a size 6, if you are put together and proportioned, the overall visual effect is the same—that is, "Hey, that's one fashionable and shapely lady!"

Bodacious Butts and Thighs

Let's look at our curvier models first to see which pants look good on them—and which ones definitely don't. Curves themselves are great, but there are good curvy looks and bad ones. (Again, it's all about being in proportion.)

This time, we'll start with Felisha. Her figure challenges in the nether regions are thicker thighs and shorter (she likes to say "stumpier") legs. She has a broad squarish torso (which is actually nicely proportionate with her broader shoulders) and a nice flat tummy. So how do we sculpt her shape? We want pants that de-emphasize her thighs and elongate her legs. What to avoid? Any pants that add girth to her hip and thigh area (with pleats, side pockets, a front zip or tab front), or a material that has bulk (like nubby wool or wide-wale corduroy).

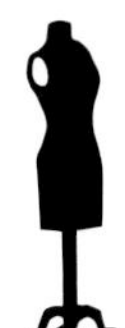

closet smarts:
CURVY

felisha before

Here we see Felisha in pants that are not working so well with her figure. The side pockets add width just where she doesn't want it, and the waist on the pants is high enough to really place some focus on the whole hip area. A pair of lower-waisted pants, which would work well with her flat tummy, will lessen the visual impact of the width of that portion of her body. The pants are also made of a wool bouclé, which adds unwanted girth. (A slicker fabric with some stretch would work much better.) Though slightly flared at the bottom, which will help proportion her hips, the pants are too short, so they don't help elongate Felisha's leg. Elongating the appearance of a leg is a huge boon to proportioning out the hip and thigh area for anyone 5'8" or below (and that's most of us) and works best with the extra help of a little heel.

felisha now

A much better look for Felisha. These **SHAPE-HUGGING PANTS**, though perhaps counterintuitive for someone sensitive about thigh girth, help create a **CURVY LOOK** for Felisha on the bottom that, because it is **WELL PROPORTIONED**, does not overemphasize her thicker parts, but actually makes them work *for her*. The **STRETCH PANTS WORK WONDERS** to smooth out lumps and bumps. This version, which is **LOW-WAISTED**, de-emphasizes her hips and incorporates her thighs in a more balanced way. It's boot-legged, evening out the hip and ankle proportion. Now we see the kind of curves that are **REALLY SEXY**, not really scary! The extra length of the pants, extended with a heel, elongates Felisha's leg to keep her from looking stubby and really helps proportion out the curviness of the look. She keeps the overall **SLEEK LOOK** together with a **FORMFITTING SWEATER**, which she can get away with because of her **FLAT TUMMY**.

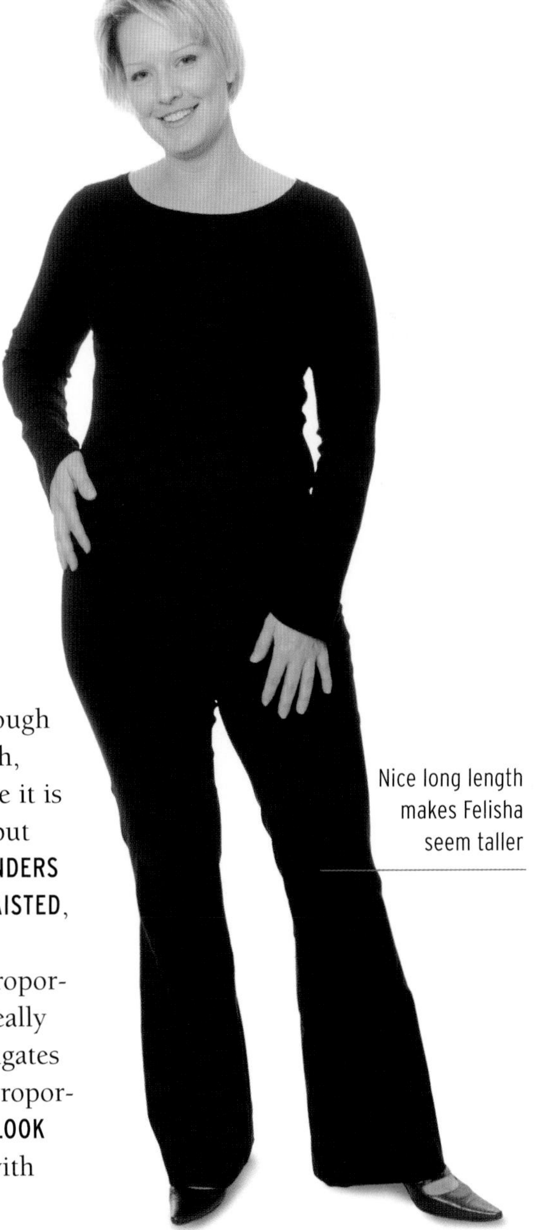

Nice long length makes Felisha seem taller

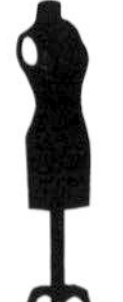

closet smarts:
CURVY

Now, let's take a look at Lily. Where pants are concerned, Lily is worried about her thighs, knees, and calves, and she also has trouble with her tummy area. She is curvy, but she tends to dress to cover over her curves, which she feels are too large, rather than accentuate them or reveal them. She has worn tapered pants in the past, which she feels draw attention to a slim ankle, and she tends to cover her top half with bigger shirts and jackets.

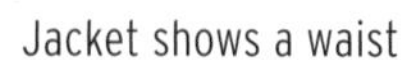
Jacket shows a waist

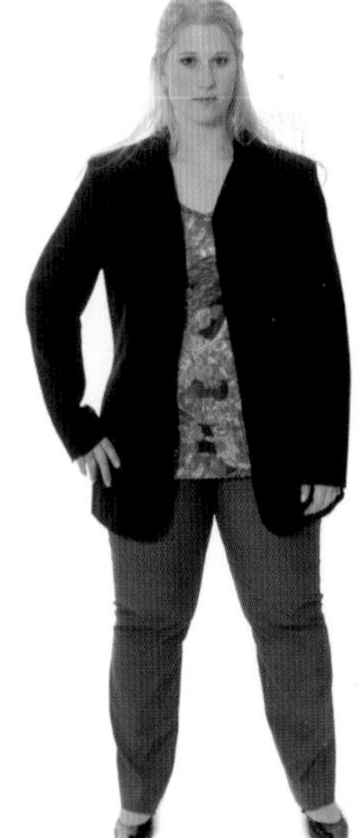

lily before

Lily has done herself a disservice here, as the tapered pants really end up emphasizing the width of her thigh and hip area, and the oversized jacket and shirt make her top half look bigger and boxier than it is as well. As I mentioned earlier, here's a case where showing more of herself rather than covering up would make Lily actually look smaller.

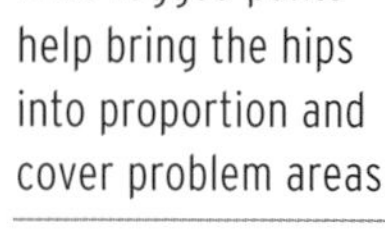
Wide-legged pants help bring the hips into proportion and cover problem areas

lily now

Here's Lily in better-suited pants and top. Again, we put her in **STRETCH PANTS** that both **HUG HER FIGURE** and **SLIM AND SMOOTH** over any lumps and bumps. In addition to the smooth appearance caused by the stretchy fabric, the shape of the pants (medium-waisted, flat-fronted, wide-legged, and long) helps skim over Lily's hips and thighs and elongate her lower half (with the help of a **REFINED HEEL**). She wears a stretchy oxford shirt that nicely masks any tummy problems and smoothes over the front of her pants. And she crisps the look up with a **SMART JACKET** that keeps the entire outfit in proportion.

Yvette also worries about the girth of her hips and thighs, though overall, she has a well-proportioned body like Lily. We have seen her in previous chapters in some great suited looks that really work, but here is another pants option for these figure challenges: the palazzo pant.

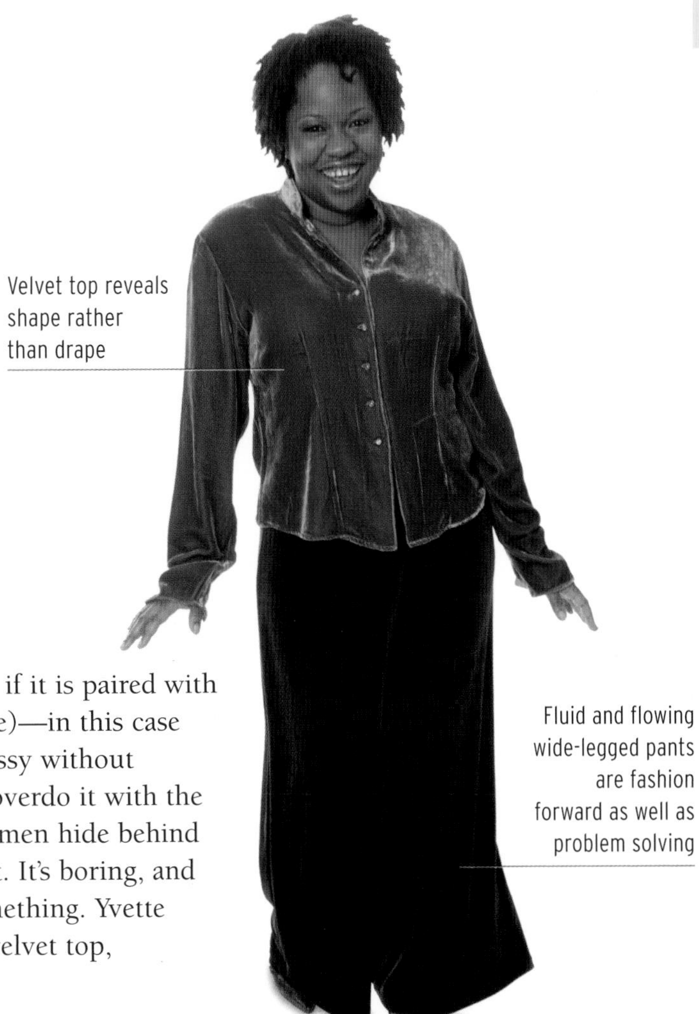

Velvet top reveals shape rather than drape

Fluid and flowing wide-legged pants are fashion forward as well as problem solving

yvette now

A pair of **FLUID WIDE-LEGGED PANTS**, especially if it is paired with a top that has some shape (rather than drape)—in this case some **GOOD FRONT DARTS**—can look really classy without looking too big. One caveat, though: Don't overdo it with the black velvet thing. I have seen too many women hide behind the monochromatic flowy black velvet outfit. It's boring, and it truly looks like you are trying to hide something. Yvette **JAZZES THINGS UP** here with a vibrant green velvet top, and she looks **SASSY, NOT FRUMPY**.

Pants with tapered legs do nothing for anyone but emphasize hips disproportionately!

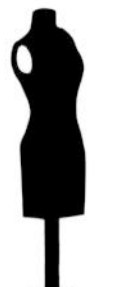

closet smarts:
CURVY

Beth has got big hips *and* a big butt to contend with. Let's consider two photos of Beth in which she is wearing pants that aren't doing her any favors, followed by two really great looks for her.

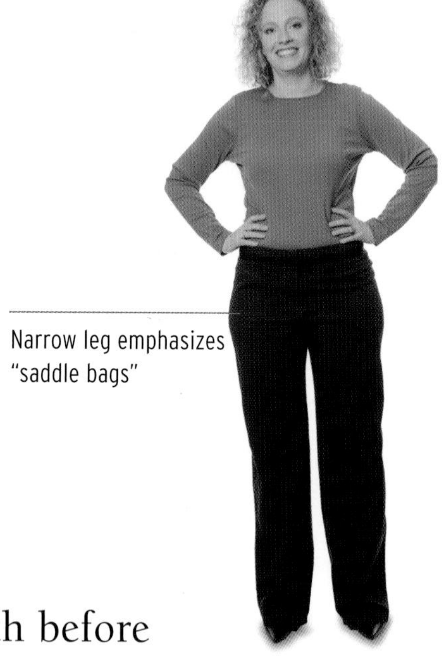

Narrow leg emphasizes "saddle bags"

beth before

These pants are pretty high-waisted, so they actually emphasize Beth's hip area and accentuate the disproportion there. What she needs is a pair of lower-rise pants that starts halfway through her hips' curve (thus de-emphasizing their width) paired with a longer shirt (or jacket!) to cover the belly area. These pants are also narrow through the thigh, so they *really* don't help hide the saddlebag area. Though they are nice and long and straight, Beth needs pants that are cut wider through the leg as well as through the hem to keep her hips in proportion to the rest of her figure.

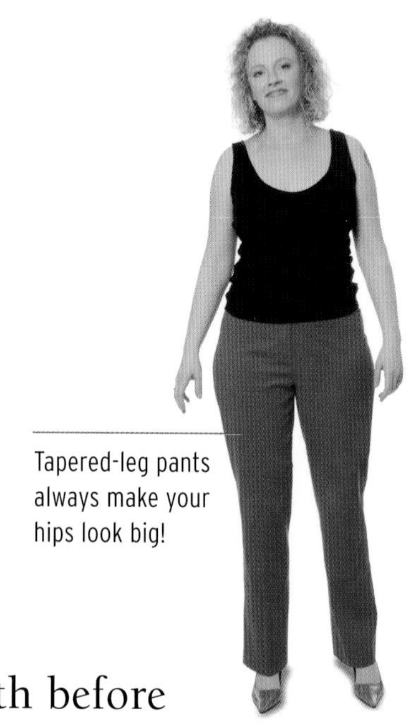

Tapered-leg pants always make your hips look big!

beth before

Tapered pants are no good for Beth, either, as the taper *emphasizes* her hips rather than *integrating* them. And these flowy lines don't work so well for Beth who, unlike Yvette and Lily, has more of a problem with disproportion in the hip department, so she can't carry the look as smoothly.

beth now

We've seen Beth in the first section of this book in other pants looks that work for her as well (straight- and wide-legged pants, also lower-rise), but here, I want to emphasize again that you can **INCORPORATE CURVES** to good effect (rather than hiding them), and the resulting look is really quite **SEXY AND APPEALING**. So *learn to love your curves*!

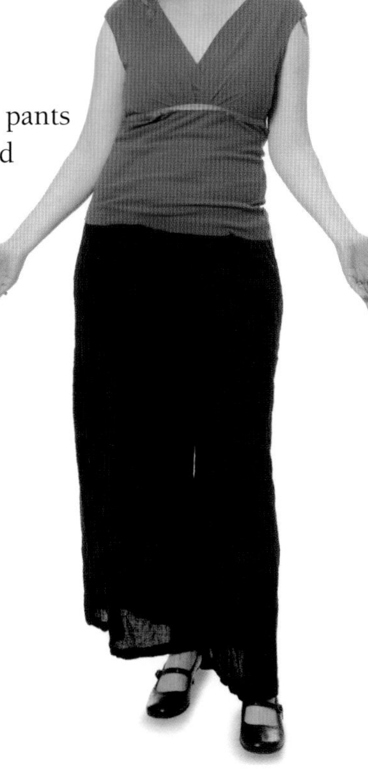

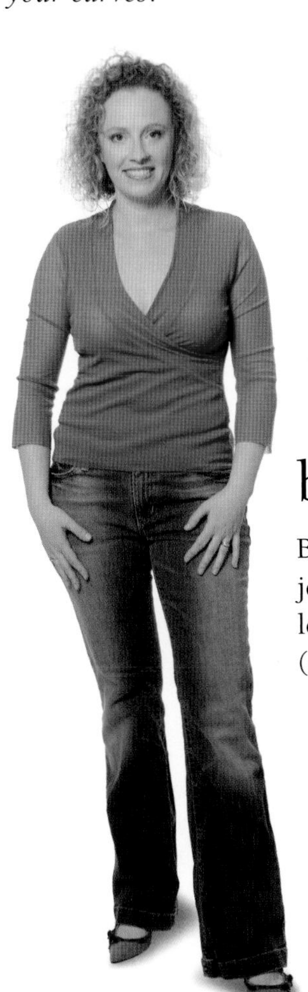

beth now

Beth's **CURVES LOOK GREAT** in these **STRETCHY**, long, boot-leg cut jeans, where the curve of her hips is evened out through the length, waist height (rise), and bootleg cut of the jean (combined, of course, with a **REFINED LOW HEEL**).

closet smarts: CURVY

For Amy, our classic hourglass, I have only one suggestion, and by now you know what it is: *Avoid tapers*!

no tapered legs!

If you have good proportions, like Amy, you'd like to keep it that way, eh? Tapers do *nothing for anyone* but emphasize hips—*disproportionately*! Please, dispense with them all immediately.

Straight and (Sometimes) Narrow

Now let's look at some of our less-curvy models and see what pants can do for—and sometimes, to—them! If your figure is straight up-and-down or you're slender (or even skinny), this section is for you.

Let's start with Karen, who has a slightly boyish figure and feels thick and straight through her lower half. A glance at the next two photos will show you why Karen should avoid pants like these:

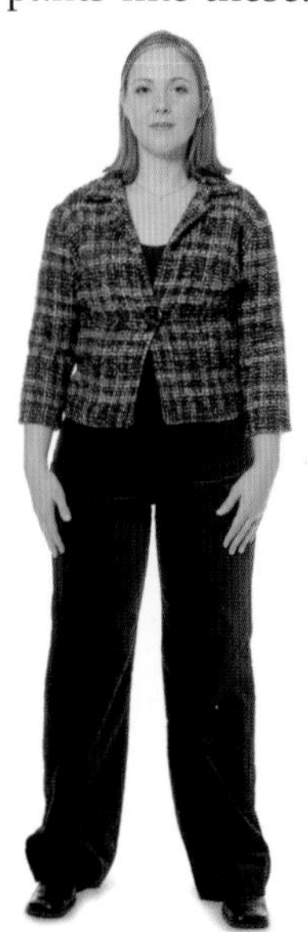

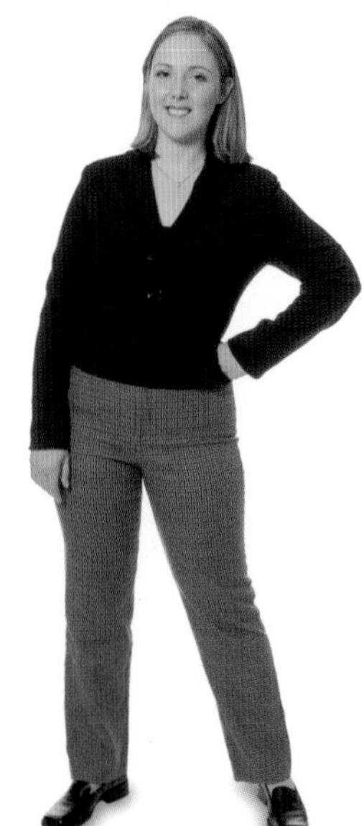

karen before

In both these cases, the pants are too high-waisted and narrow-legged, only serving to emphasize the squareness of Karen's midsection. Despite the first pairs' smoothing velveteen fabric, we get the impression from the cut of the pants that Karen is actually being *squeezed* into them, rather than *smoothed* by them. Neither look is working.

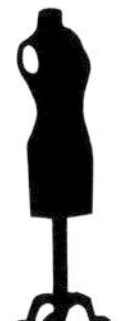

closet smarts: STRAIGHT AND NARROW

karen now

A look that really works for Karen is a lower-waisted, wider-legged pant, here combined with a formfitting sweater to really **SHOW SOME CURVES** as a counterbalance to the straighter appearance of the leg. The long, cuffed pants with a heel add a lot of height to Karen's look as well, so she avoids looking stubby and thick and instead looks **TALL AND CURVACEOUS**. What a difference!

The flow of these wide-legged pants creates a smoother silhouette

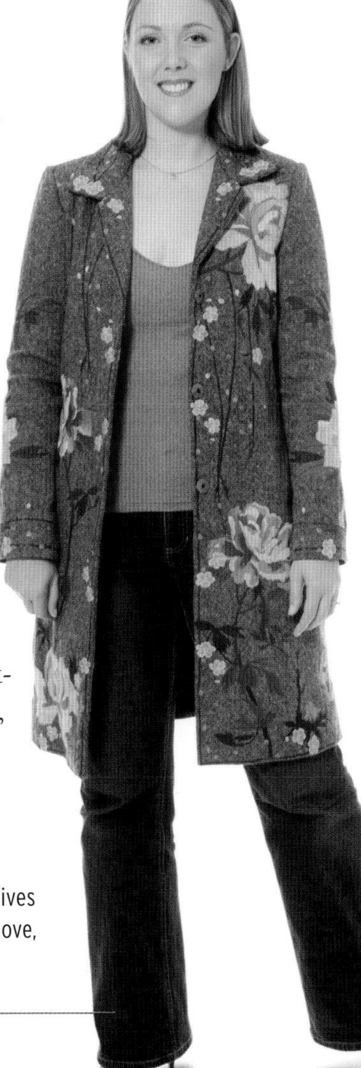

karen now

Karen also **LOOKS GREAT** in a straight-legged, **LOW-WAISTED** dark wash jean, as seen here with a **FORMFITTING TOP** and embroidered duster jacket.

Slight flare cut gives Karen room to move, plus elongates her legs

closet smarts:
STRAIGHT AND NARROW

Supriya will provide us with our lesson about pleated pants. Here goes: Please, please, never *ever* wear pleated pants, no matter what your figure type! If anyone could use some girth about the midsection, it's Supriya, but this is *not* the way to go!

We've seen Supriya in a number of great pants looks throughout the first half of the book, and here is another that works for her figure.

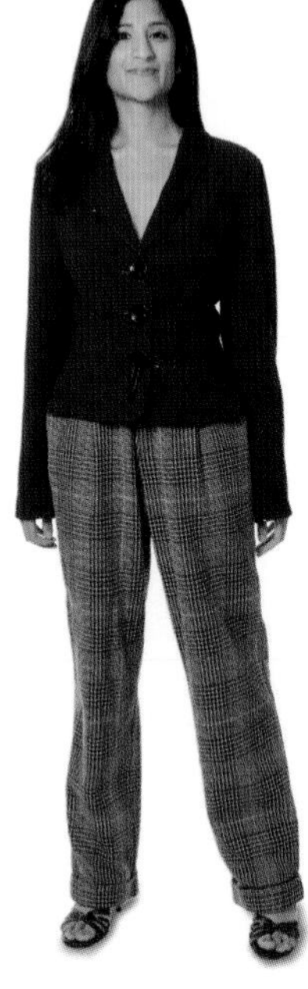

supriya before

As far as I am concerned, these are clown pants. Pleats automatically draw attention to that part of the torso most women are dying to distract you from—the "pooch" —and they actually help create the illusion that you have *more* of a pooch than you may actually have. On Supriya, they just make these pants seem ill-fitting on her slight frame, and combined with their subtler taper, create the dreaded pencil silhouette we've all been working studiously hard to avoid since reading chapter 7 (right?). Again, Supriya would like to add a little shapeliness to her bottom half, and perhaps some height, but none of that is being accomplished here.

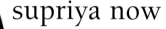

supriya now

Though Supriya can afford to wear higher-waisted pants with her long torso, with this **BABYDOLL** top, it doesn't matter much and these lower-rise pants suit her well. They're **SLIM-FITTING** so as not to overwhelm her skinnier legs, but still **FLARED** at the bottom to both keep her shoulders in **PROPORTION** and to counter-balance her skinniness. The longer pants leg paired with a heel also add height to her appearance, which is **ALWAYS A BOON** in proportion science.

Length combined with heel really adds length and height to Supriya's look

Narrow-legged pants don't overwhelm skinnier legs

On Deborah, who is even skinner than Supriya, we use a more extreme flared pant to add a little width to her overall silhouette and to balance out her shoulders.

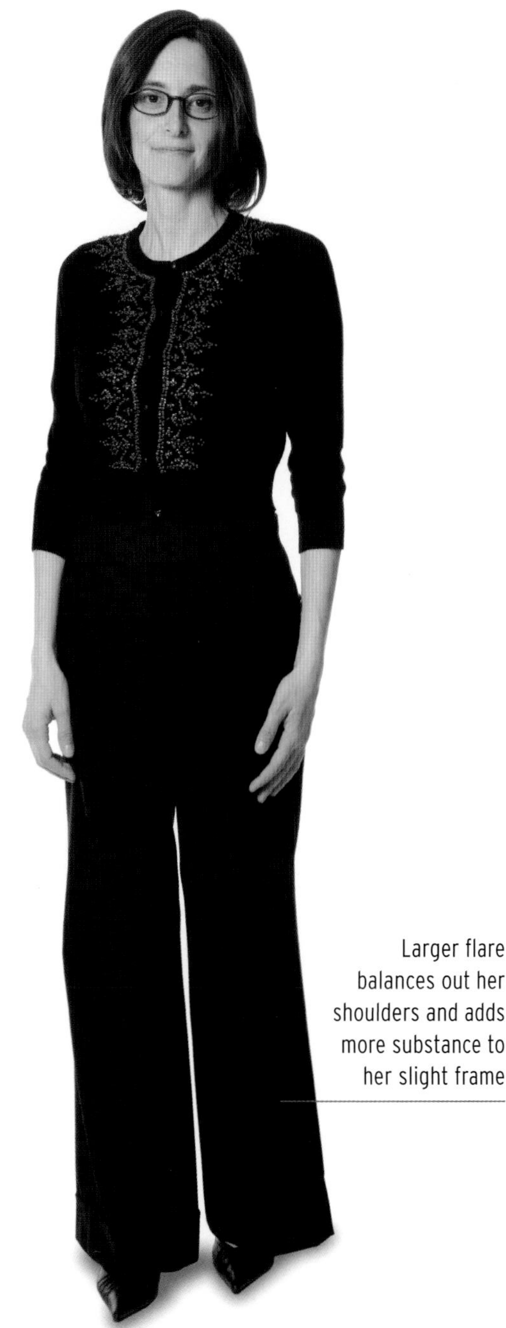

deborah now

In addition to putting Deborah in flared pants, the **LAYERING** of her sweater and top also **ADDS SOME SHAPE** to her slight frame and helps **CREATE SOME CURVES** at the waist and bust.

Larger flare balances out her shoulders and adds more substance to her slight frame

Long and Leggy

And what about our tall gal Morgan, who is concerned about her oversized booty and womanly hips? Check out the photos below, and you'll see three wrong looks. They actually call attention to Morgan's heavy area—finally hitting the right one (next page).

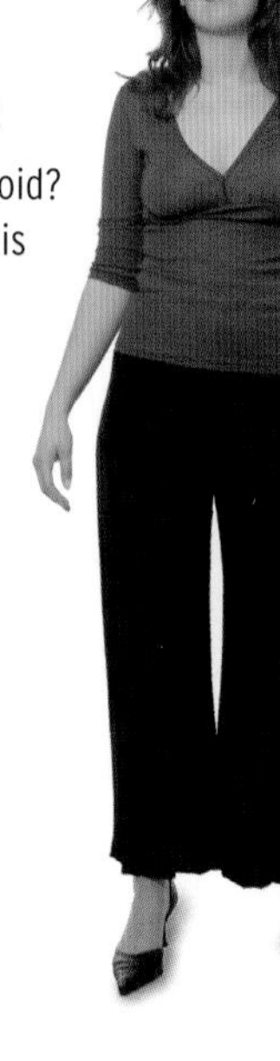

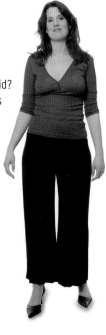

morgan before

What else should Morgan avoid? Fluid and flowy pants like this will accentuate the size and shape of her hips.

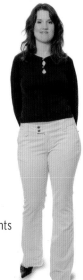

morgan before

First and foremost, Morgan should avoid higher-waisted, slim-fitting pants like these. They only draw attention to her butt and accentuate it.

morgan before

Another tip? Side pockets, even on wider-legged pants styles, are no good for Morgan, as they also draw attention to and exacerbate the trouble zone.

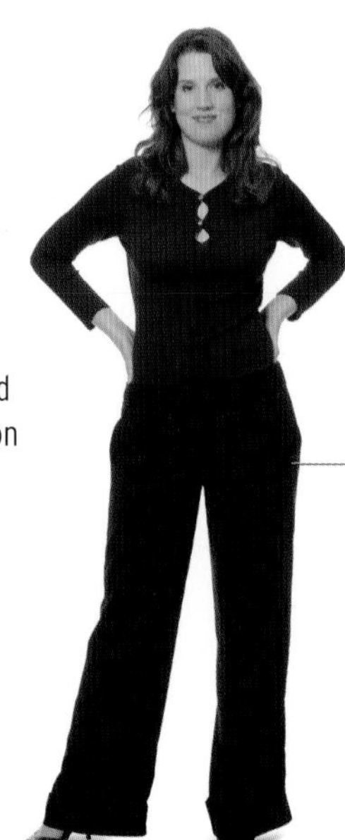

Side pockets add girth where she doesn't want it

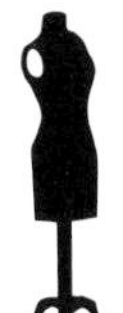

closet smarts:
TALL

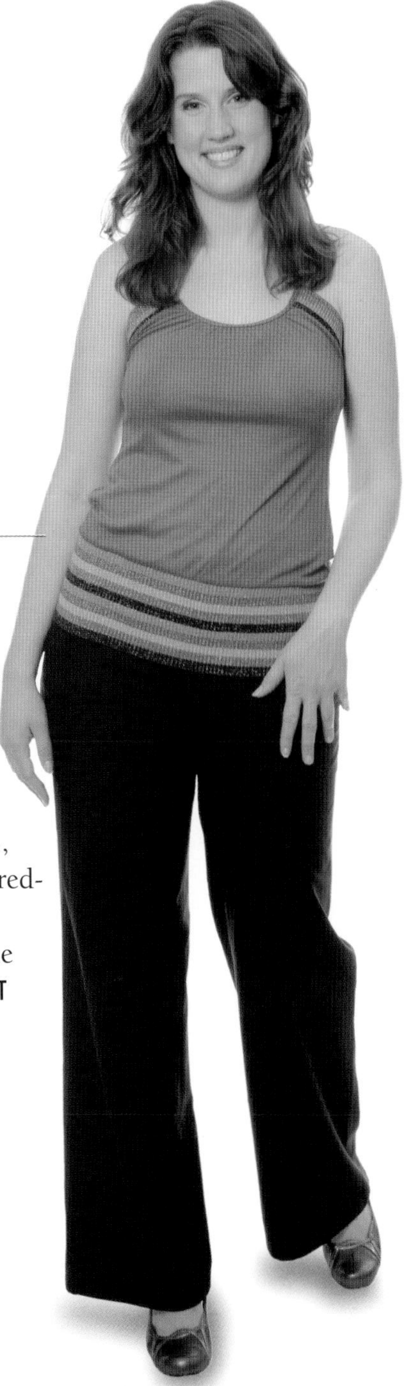

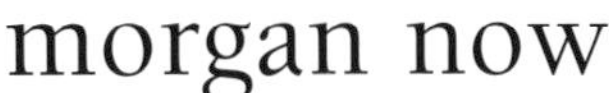

morgan now

So what works for Morgan? For this **GORGEOUS**, leggy Amazon, a pair of simple straight- or flared-leg pants, lower-waisted and flat-fronted, and preferably in a **FIRMER FABRIC** to smooth out the derriere and thighs, is the way to go. She **CAN'T MISS** with this look!

The Last Word

Okay, *now* do you believe there are great pants looks for every body, even yours? Have you seen yourself in some of the photos in this chapter, and maybe even said, "She's right. I have pants like that"? Remember, ladies, the Goodwill is waiting. Do your bottom half—and your bottom—a big favor and take those tapered, high-waisted, and/or pleated horrors to a galaxy far, far away. Then buy yourself some pants that look really *good*. You've seen living proof that pants will look good on you. So get out there and try them on!

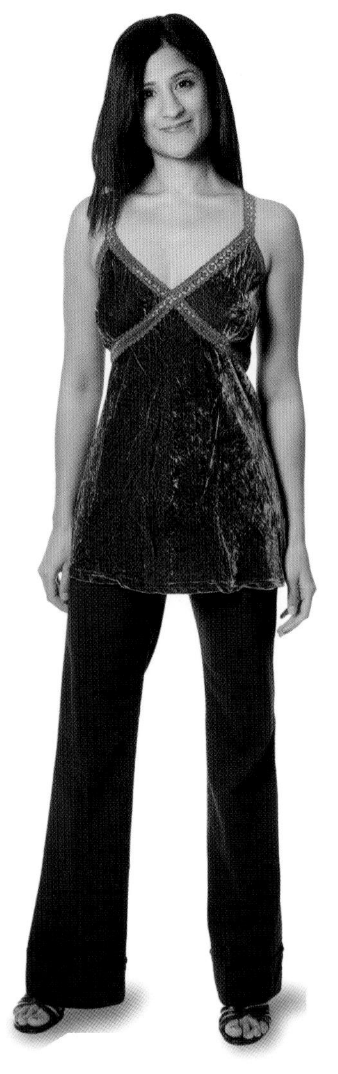

Pants will *look good on you.*

So, you've seen the pants tricks, and they are pretty consistent across the board if you keep two things in mind: the goal of proportioning and the two-triangle model (create the waist and keep the top and bottom ends proportionate). Pretty simple, eh? How does the same strategy look when applied to skirts? In the next chapter, we will explore good and bad skirt looks for our models, and hopefully for *you*.

ULTIMATE PANTS STYLE

Whether you're trying to minimize your curves or enhance them, or just show off that perfect hourglass shape, remember these tips, and you'll know what to look for and what to avoid at all costs.

1. Hips are *emphasized* by a high-waisted pant. If you have larger hips, try pants that start about halfway down your hip line and combine them with a longer top to avoid belly exposure for your best look.
2. Narrow-legged pants call attention to hips and thighs. A pair of wider boot-cut, straight-cut, or even palazzo pants evens out the figure and slenderizes the leg.
3. Pants with tapered legs don't flatter anybody, whatever their figure.
4. Pleats are a big no-no. They only draw attention to the undesirable "pooch"—something we'd all like to forget about, not emphasize.
5. Wearing heels with your pants always helps elongate the leg and gives you a sleeker, more put-together look.

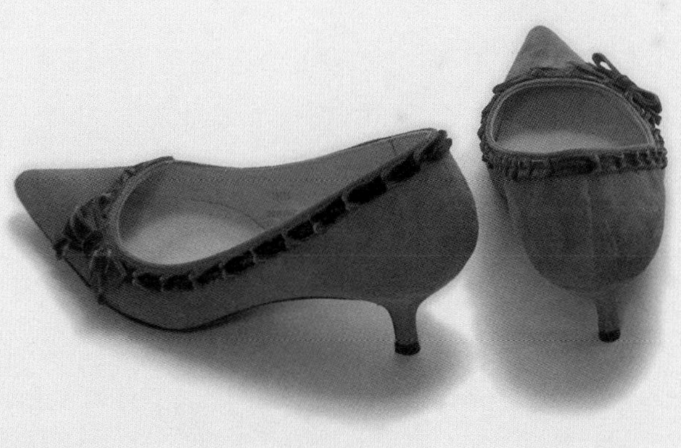

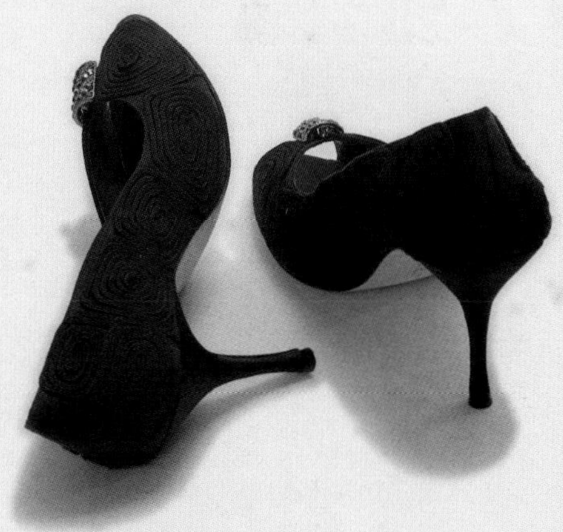

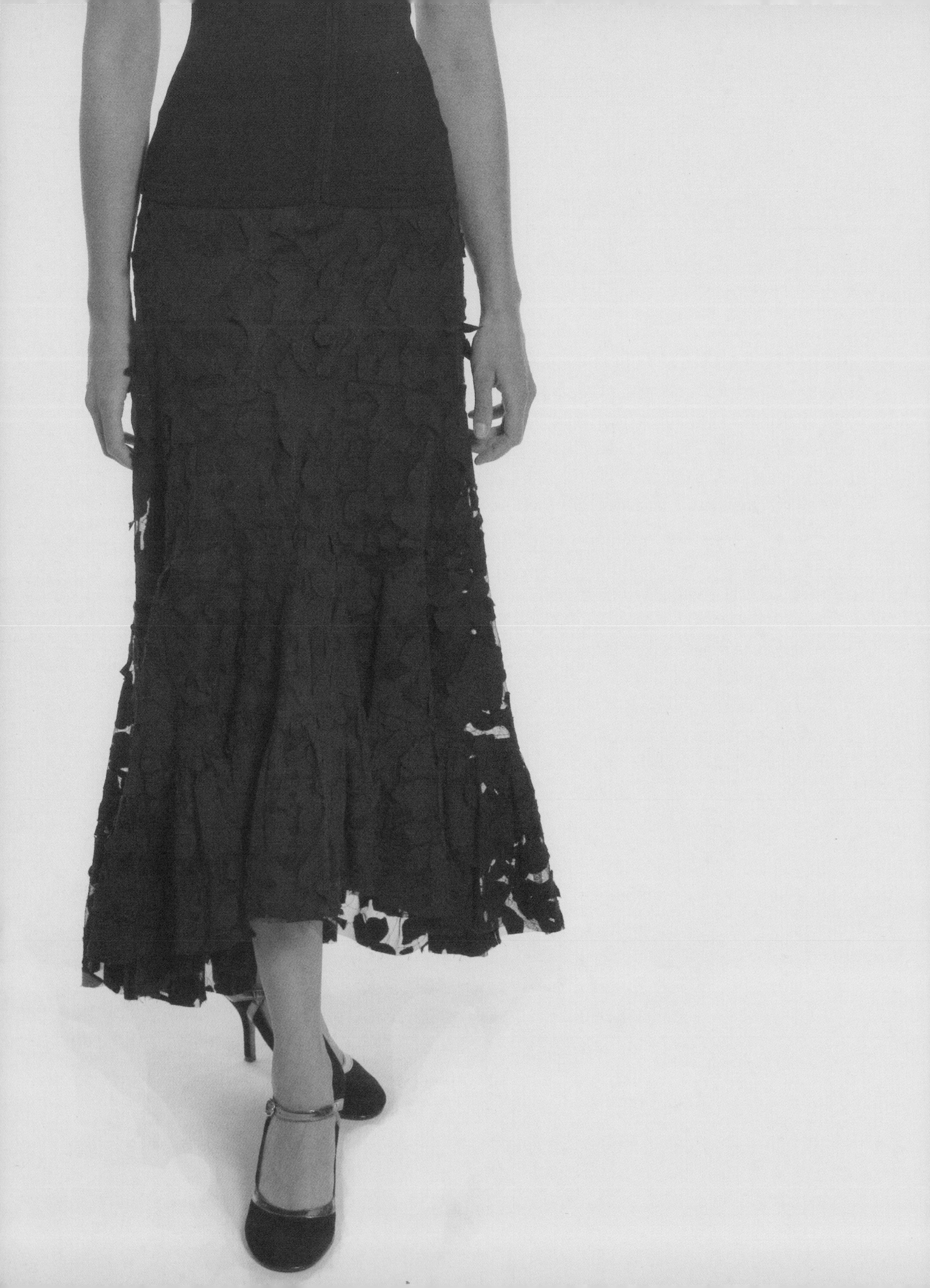

CHAPTER 9

skirting the issue

Lines, Lengths, and (Great-Looking) Legs

9

When talking about skirts—or wearing them, as the case may be—there are certain basic things you have to think about: What length is appropriate for you? What basic shape would look best? What design details enhance or detract from your shape? You'll find all the answers in this chapter. Much like the last, we'll use our models' figures as guides, and we'll find solutions for *your* figure along the way!

Though the issues here are similar to pants issues when it comes to hips and tummies, a skirt is a skirt, not a pair of pants. With skirts, the cuts are basically pencil, A-line, straight, fluted, flared/flowy, and bias-cut. The lengths are above the knee, knee-length, mid-calf, and ankle. The design details are slits, ruffles, asymmetric hems, tiers, gathers, yokes, pleats, and belts. The fabrics are too many to name. So you see, we won't be skirting the issues here! Rather, as we tackle skirts head-on, keep in mind our mantras about proportion, silhouette, and the Two-Triangle Theory. They will get you through your darkest fashion moments.

Battling Our Biases and Other Full-Figured Pitfalls

Ready to look at some skirts? We'll start again with Felisha, who agonizes over her "thick" thighs when getting dressed in the morning.

CLOSET SMARTS STYLE: DON'T BE BIASED

A bias-cut skirt, which is a fairly common cut, is cut diagonally across the fabric, giving it a natural cling about the hips and usually narrowing about the ankles. For larger-hipped women, this spells D-I-S-A-S-T-E-R. Avoid these skirts like the plague! Most of them are made in silk fabric anyway and tend to bunch at the hemline and on the hips (adding insult to injury), so you really don't need to be bothering with these. Leave 'em for the skinny Minnies who don't have hips. Instead, if you have big hips, look for A-line skirts. An A-line naturally flares away from the hips, creating a smooth line over potential trouble zones.

If you have big hips look for A-line skirts.

felisha before

A big no-no for Felisha is a bias-cut skirt like she's wearing in this photo. The cling of a skirt like this just makes her hips look bigger. Felisha's best bet (as is true for *most* figures, believe it or not) is an A-line skirt, as you'll see in the next two photos.

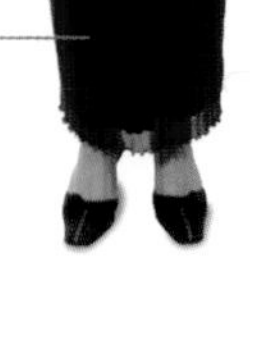

Clinging at the hips is not good when you want proportion

Narrow bottom of bias is like tapered pants—not good!

closet smarts:
FULL-FIGURE PITFALLS

felisha now

This skirt sits low on Felisha's waist (another trick for de-emphasizing the width of the hip zone that you may remember from the pants chapter). The **LOW-WAISTED DETAILING** is accentuated by her low-slung sash. The vertical seaming throughout the skirt helps **ELONGATE** her lower half as well, so we are not stuck with the stocky thick Felisha, but rather we are left with the impression of a **GRACEFULLY FLOWING** Felisha.

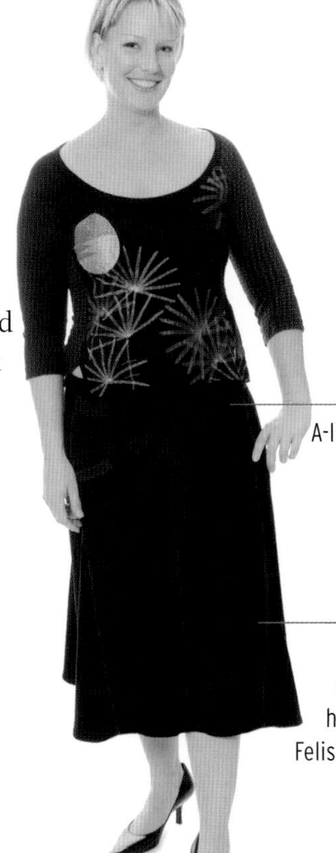

A-line completely covers her hip troubles

Longer length combined with heels elongates Felisha's silhouette

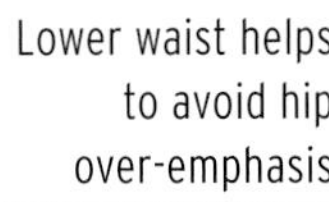

Lower waist helps to avoid hip over-emphasis

felisha now

Here's **ANOTHER GREAT LOOK** for Felisha, a longer (mid-calf), slightly flared denim skirt. The A-line here distracts the eye from any hip issues, and the stiffer denim **SMOOTHES OVER** the lumps and bumps. But there's more: The mid-calf length, when combined with a refined heel, has the effect of **ELONGATING** Felisha's lower half and making her look **TALLER**.

Vertical seams help to elongate the look

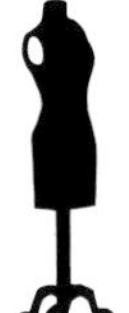

closet smarts:
FULL-FIGURE PITFALLS

Lily, who is more curvy all over, has a different set of issues. Let's look at her options.

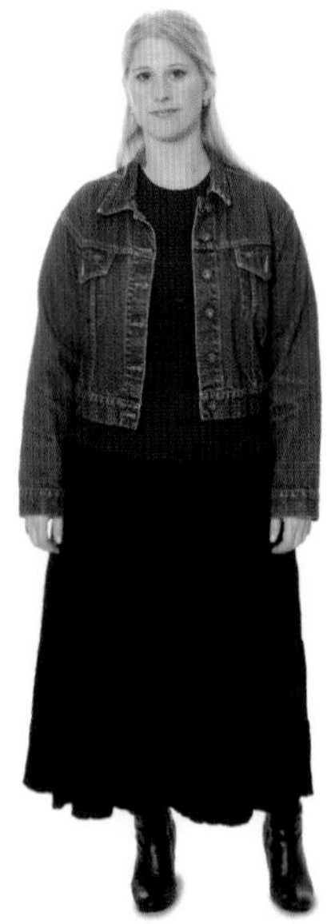

lily before

Lily is tempted to cover up with this extra-flowy ankle-length number. No way! Lily has some much better skirting options, as you can see from the next group of photos.

Formfitting top emphasizes her shapeliness at the waist and bust, while wrap top contains the tummy

lily now

First, Lily could try the opposite of her instincts and opt to really **SHOWCASE** her curves. In this **FLUTED SKIRT**, though her hips are emphasized by the skirt's cut, the fluted ruffle detail at the bottom really balances out the hip. Combined with a **FORMFITTING** top, which **ACCENTUATES** her curves throughout, Lily looks **REALLY SEXY** as she owns her curves while keeping them smooth and proportioned.

Fluted ruffle balances out the hips

lily now

Lily can also wear a straighter version of the **PENCIL SKIRT** to good effect, as it allows room for her hips while not overboxifying her look. It also shows off her **SHAPELY CALVES** and slim ankles. We see her here in a more fun version as well as a more work-appropriate version.

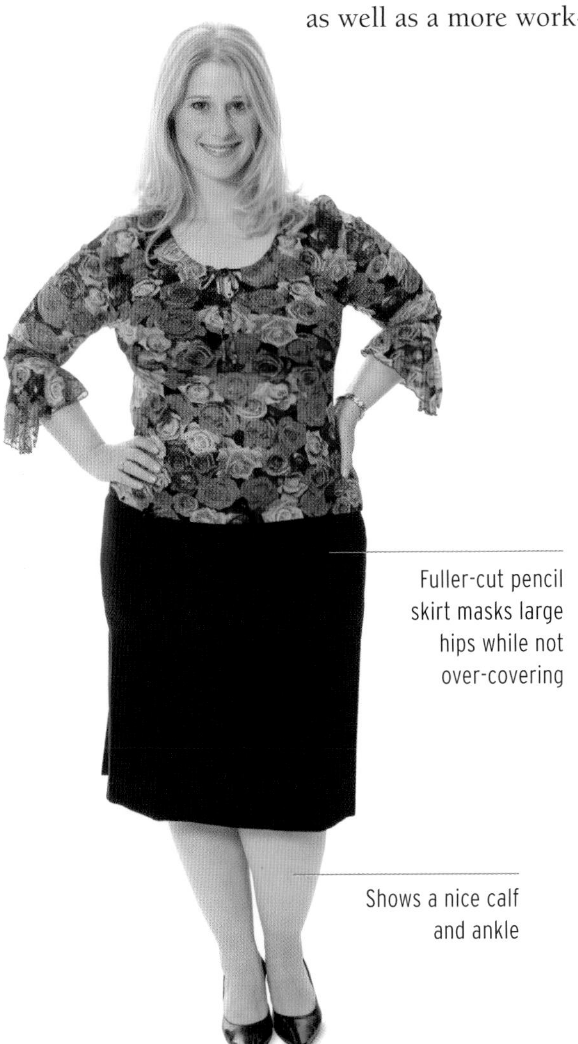

Fuller-cut pencil skirt masks large hips while not over-covering

Shows a nice calf and ankle

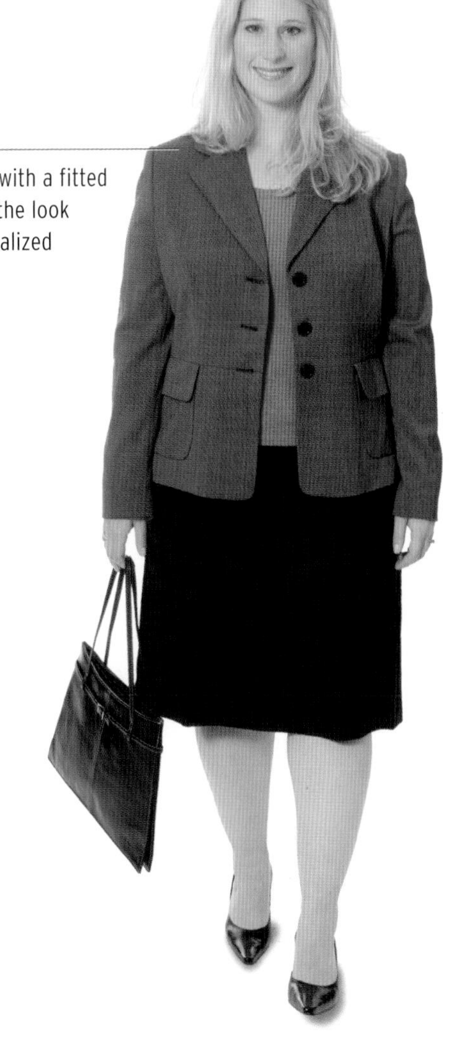

Paired with a fitted jacket the look is formalized

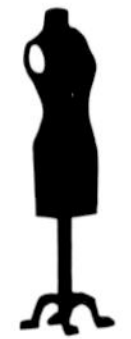

closet smarts:
FULL-FIGURE PITFALLS

Yvette seemed to embody both extremes when it came to skirt dressing: Super-short for fun, super-long for work. Neither look really works for Yvette, as you can see from the first two photos below. Her "play" look is way too young for her, though I convinced her she doesn't have to give up sexy when dressing for fun. Compare and contrast the two "after" shots on page 155 and see for yourself!

You don't have to give up sexy when dressing for fun.

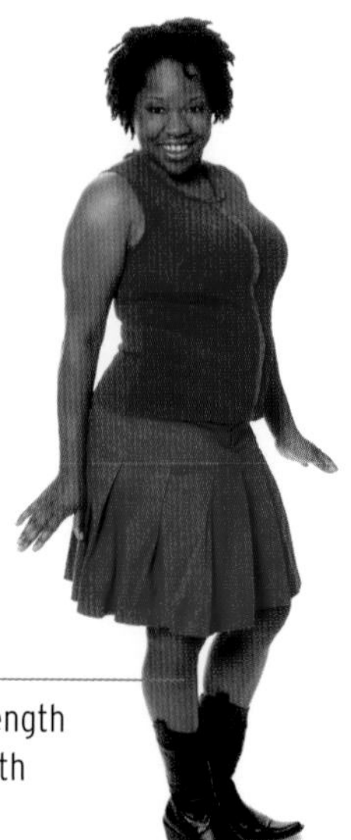

yvette before

For fun, Yvette would don this pleated miniskirt (a true Texan at heart).

Flared knee-length pleats add girth to hips

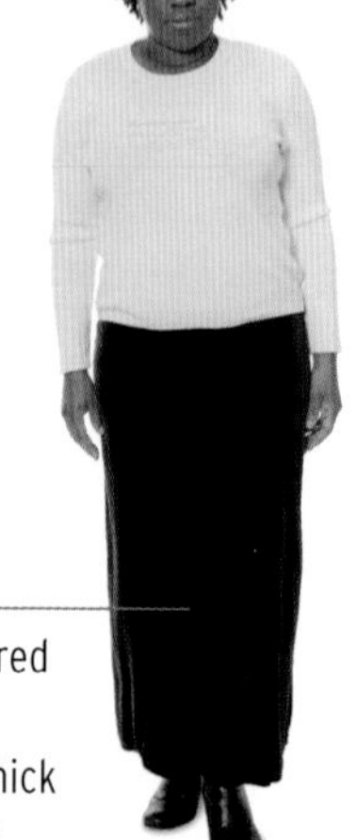

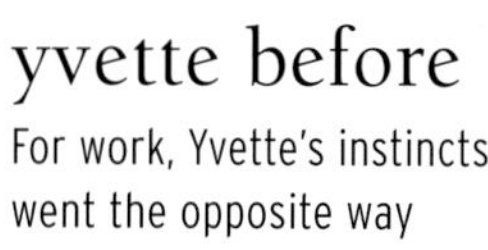

yvette before

For work, Yvette's instincts went the opposite way —take cover!

Long, unstructured skirt makes her lower half too thick and rectangular

9

yvette now

For Yvette's work look, we used this below-the-knee, slightly A-line skirt with a **RUFFLED BOTTOM** (to even out the hips) combined with a **FITTED TOP** and jacket for a **SLEEK PROFESSIONAL LOOK**. With this outfit, we get to see all the great parts—**DÉCOLLETAGE**, ankles, and calves, and yes, **GREAT CURVES**.

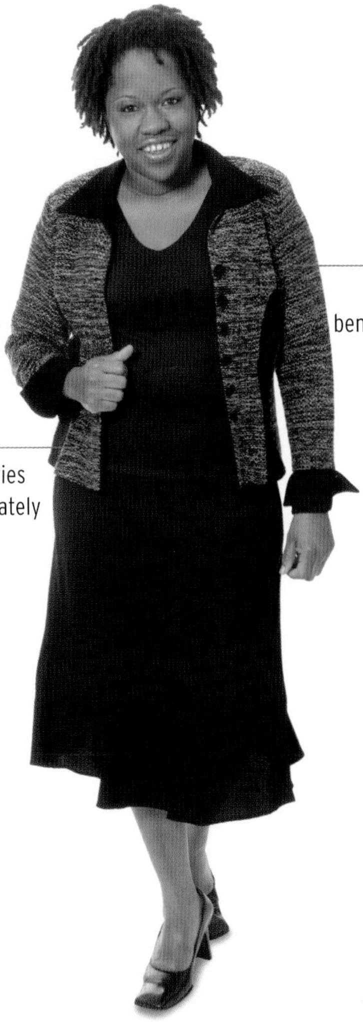

Fitted shirt beneath shows a slimmer silhouette rather than bulking up the look

Shapely jacket caries curves proportionately throughout

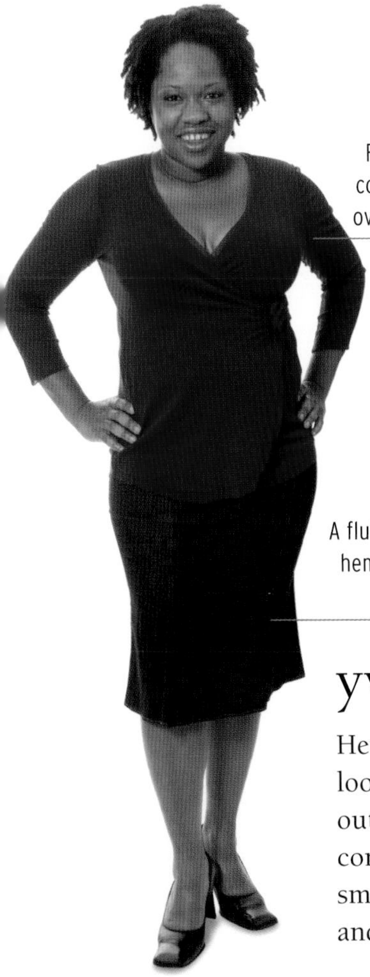

Fitted shirt adds consistency to an overall curvy look

A flute at the skirt's hem helps balance out larger hips

yvette now

Here's a **PLAY LOOK** that does work for Yvette. Like Lily's curvy look on page 152, the flute of this skirt functions to balance out Yvette's hips, and the **FITTED** shirt makes the **CURVY LOOK** consistent throughout. The denim goes a long way toward smoothing out any problem areas as well, and the empire waist and **FAUX WRAP** on top provide **NICE TUMMY COVERAGE**.

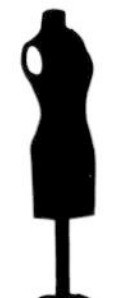

closet smarts:
FULL-FIGURE PITFALLS

Let's look now at Beth, who's concerned about ample hips and saddlebags. As you'll see, she hasn't been doing herself any favors in the skirt department.

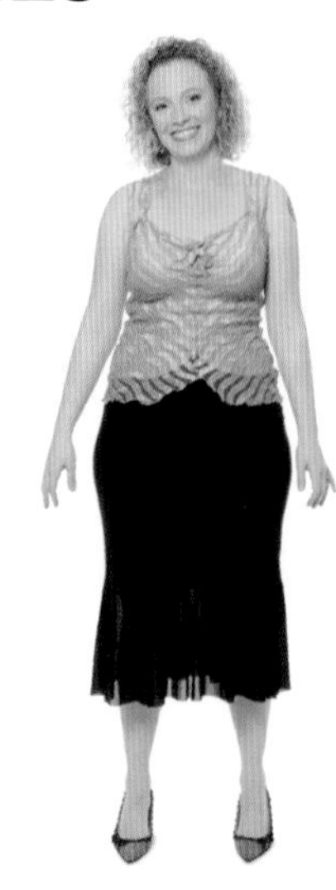

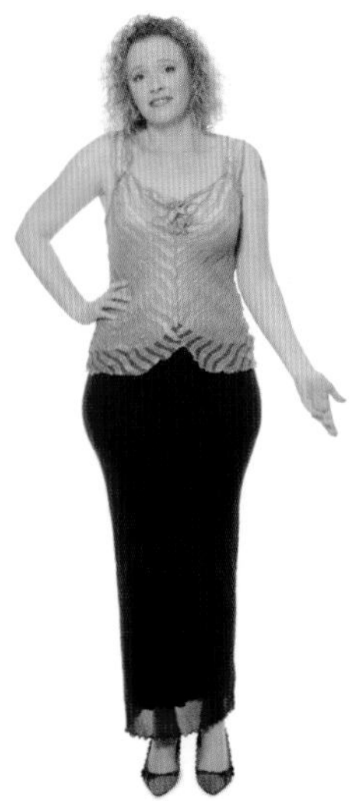

beth before

These bias-cut skirts aren't so great for the saddlebag effect, are they? Longer biases, even those with a ruffle, are no good for Beth.

CLOSET SMARTS STYLE: THE YOKE'S ON YOU

Skirts with yokes can be real friends to those of us with fuller figures. A yoke on a skirt is like an extended waistband, where the skirt fits closely to the body up to the yoke's edge and then drapes away, usually into an A-line—a great boon for skimming over troublesome hips.

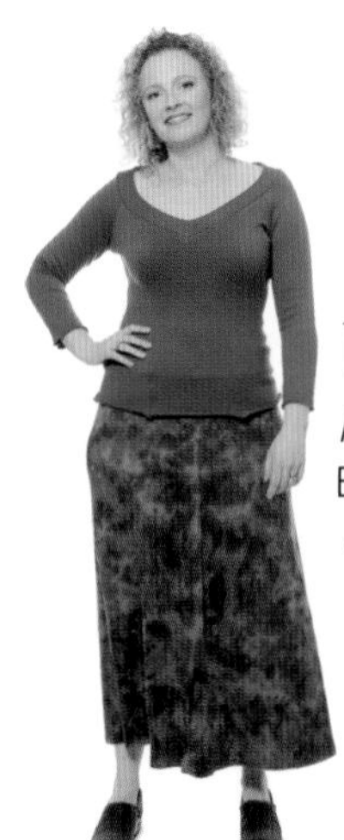

beth before

Anything longer than mid-calf on Beth really plumps her up by adding too much material to her frame, like this overly flowy ankle-length number.

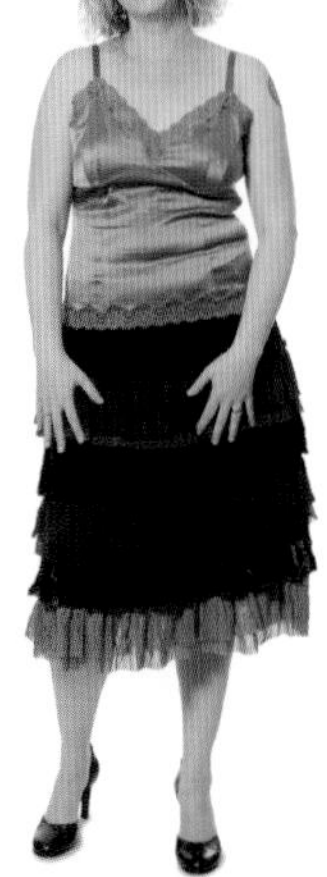

beth before

Also wrong: Design add-ons that hit at the wrong place on Beth's hip zone, emphasizing girth, like this tiered skirt.

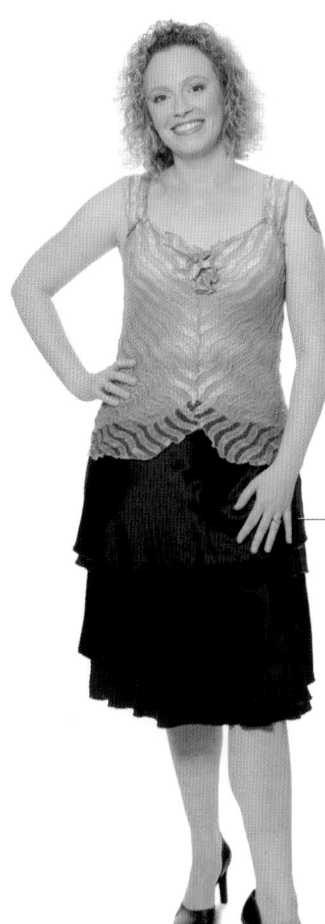

beth now

However, skirts with **A YOKE** long enough to make it past Beth's trouble zone before breaking out into a **DESIGN** (in this case a tier) **CAN REALLY WORK** to de-emphasize her hips' width.

This tier hits at the right place, smoothing over her hips

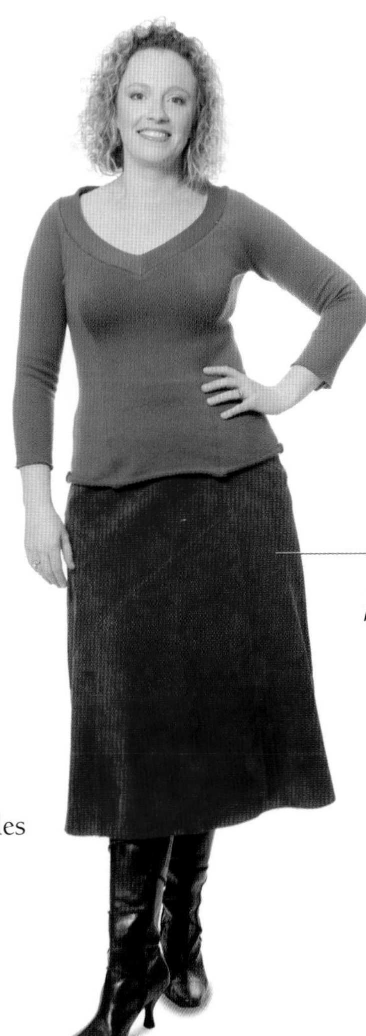

The beauty of the A-line, it smoothes over everything!

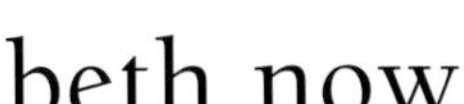

beth now

Beth **LOOKS BEST** in knee- to mid-calf-length skirts. Though we have seen her in a number of different styles throughout the book, her **SUREFIRE SKIRT** shape is an A-line like this. **ALWAYS FLATTERING**!

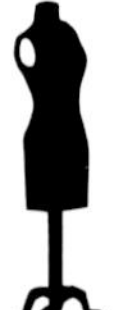

closet smarts: HOURGLASS FIGURE

What about Amy, our hourglass girl? Even a girl with great proportions can pick the wrong skirt, as Amy did in the first two photos below.

amy before

See what I mean? A bias cut = no good for hips, even well-proportioned hips like Amy's!

Bias=bad for hips

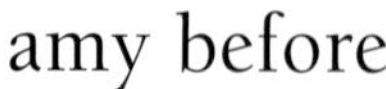

amy before

This full-bodied knee-length skirt also does nothing for Amy's figure: The length is all wrong. It's too young-looking, and it cuts her body at an awkward place for the overall silhouette. (She ends up looking short.) Even worse, its width makes her look stumpy rather than curvy or svelte.

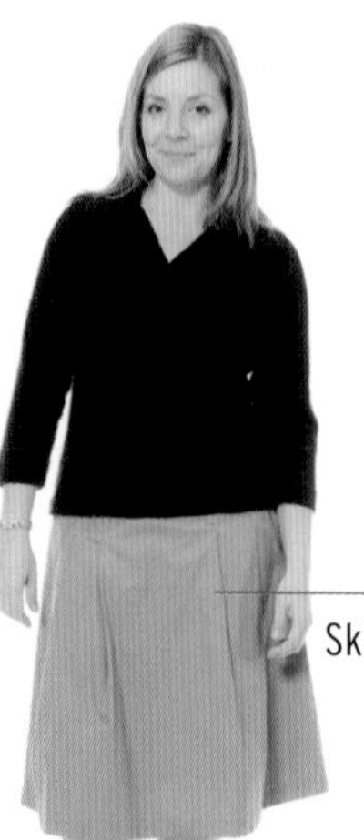

Skirt hits at her widest part

amy now

Amy looks much **LEANER AND LONGER** in this mid-calf denim skirt with its **GRACEFUL A-LINE** shape. Its length is **MORE SOPHISTICATED** for Amy, and it even makes her look **TALLER**. We've seen Amy in several other photos throughout the book **LOOKING GREAT** in an A-line as well.

3/4 length elongates Amy's silhouette

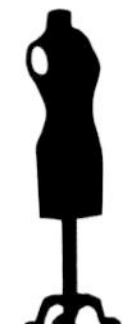

closet smarts: ADDING PROPORTION

Sara, whose stature is close to Amy's but whose figure is less curvy overall, has similar trouble with knee-length flared skirts.

sara before

This knee-length flared skirt just ends up chopping Sara at an awkward place and making her look wider than she actually is. The look, again, is too girlish, despite the lace overlay. For someone who worries about being too squarish and broad on the top, a softer, curvier look is what we should cultivate in Sara's skirting.

sara now

Another, more **CASUAL**, skirted look that works on Sara's squarish figure is this fluted denim stretch (read **CURVE-HUGGING**) skirt. Combined with a top with rounded shoulders that help **SOFTEN** her own, while its empire waist and **DEEP V-NECK** accentuate the curve of her bust, there is nothing square about this look. Sara looks great!

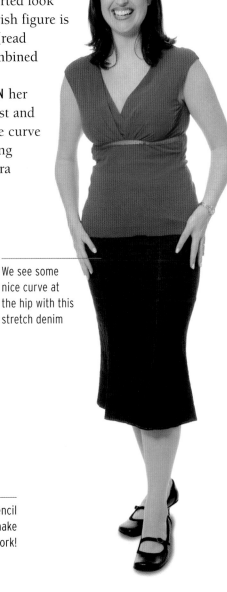

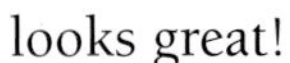

We see some nice curve at the hip with this stretch denim

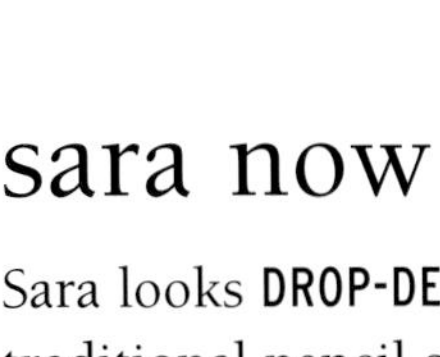

sara now

Sara looks **DROP-DEAD SEXY** in this traditional pencil skirt. It shows the curve of her hip as well as some good leg, combined here with a **FORMFITTING SWEATER** that **KEEPS THE CURVES GOING** throughout her silhouette.

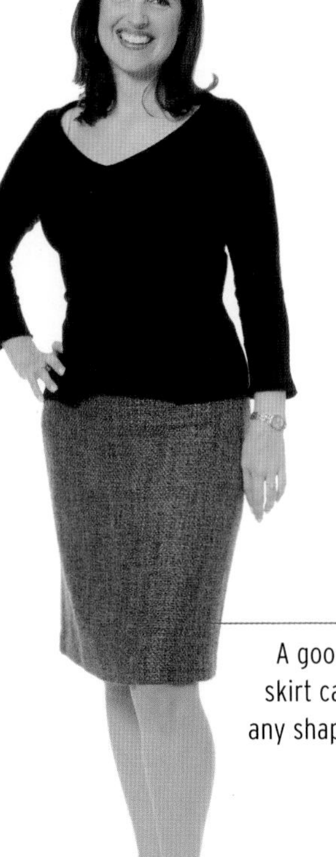

A good pencil skirt can make any shape work!

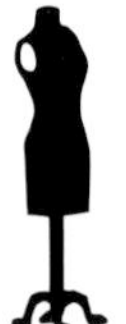

closet smarts:
BOXY BOTTOM HALF

As for Karen, who feels squarish and boxy on her bottom half, we can quickly soften her up with an A-line skirt like the two on the next page.

karen before

Where can Karen go wrong? When she adds too much fabric around her hips, making her look wider, and too much length to her skirt, making her look shorter. No good!

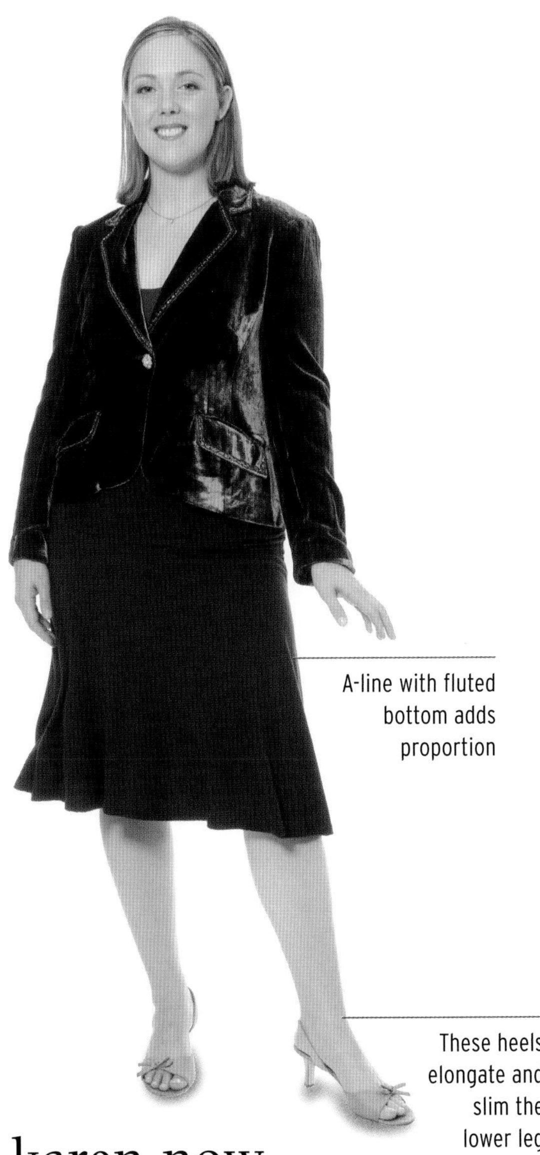

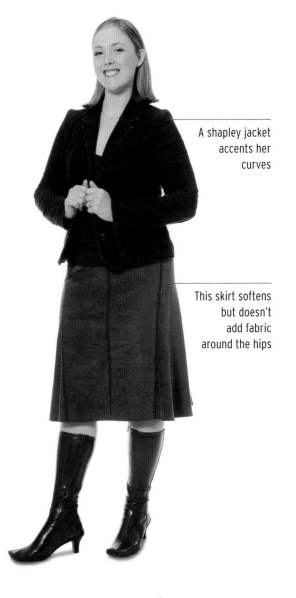

A-line with fluted bottom adds proportion
These heels elongate and slim the lower leg

A shapley jacket accents her curves
This skirt softens but doesn't add fabric around the hips

karen now

Either of these **FLUID A-LINE LOOKS** successfully skirt Karen's thighs and hips. A-line styling really seems to work for most of us, whatever our figure flaws. You should try one!

closet smarts:
SLIGHTER FRAMES

Skirts for Slighter Frames

Our slighter-framed models have different problems, but problems nonetheless. Let Supriya and Deborah show you what works—and what doesn't—for the skinny girls.

Supriya, whose has plenty of curves up top but is pretty skinny down below, could stand to add some curves and a little girth, but she has to be careful not to overwhelm her frame or end up looking too scrawny. Let's start with some unsuccessful looks, then move on to a great solution.

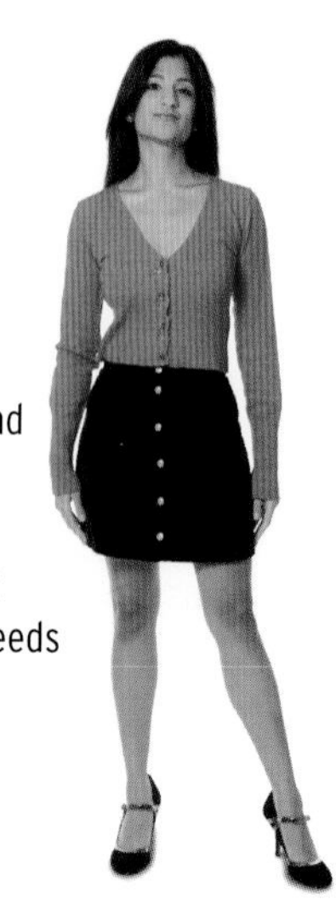

supriya before

This time, the skirt is too wide and bell-like. Supriya's legs look like they could swing back and forth like a clock's pendulum. The skirt makes them look scrawny. She needs a more fitted option.

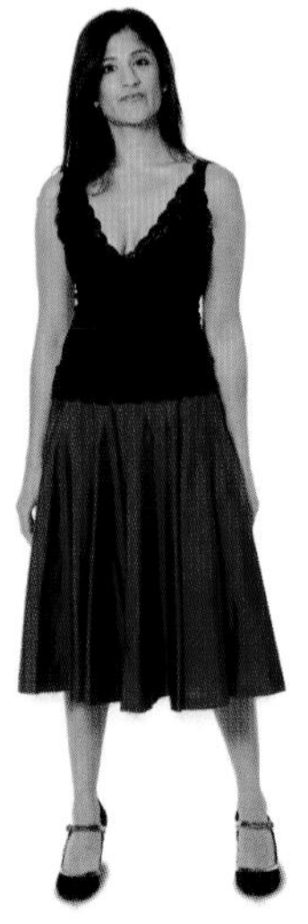

supriya before

This skirt is just too full for Supriya's small frame!

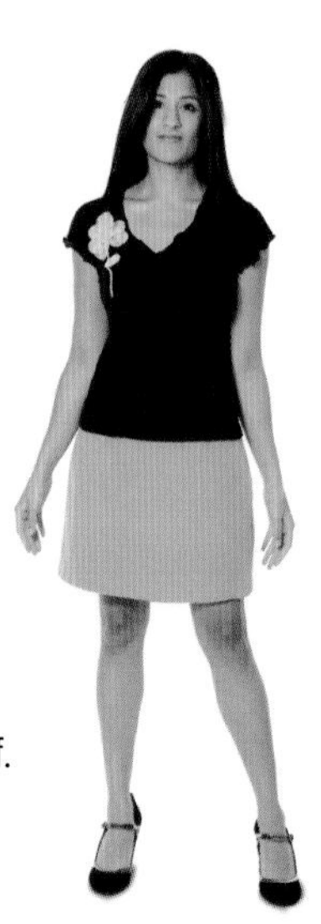

supriya before

Still not right! This time it's too short. Supriya looks too girlish here, not sexy and sophisticated, and the waistline chops her in half.

supriya now

Aaah—now here is a skirt I can get behind for Supriya. It is **SLIM-FITTING** enough to **SHOW HER SHAPE** (and add a little for that matter), but not so full as to overwhelm her. Its **CUT-OUT APPLIQUÉ** adds just the right amount of girth to her slight frame, and its flared bottom, paired with a very formfitting (read **BUST-HUGGING**) top, actually helps balance out her proportions in that department. **PERFECTO**!

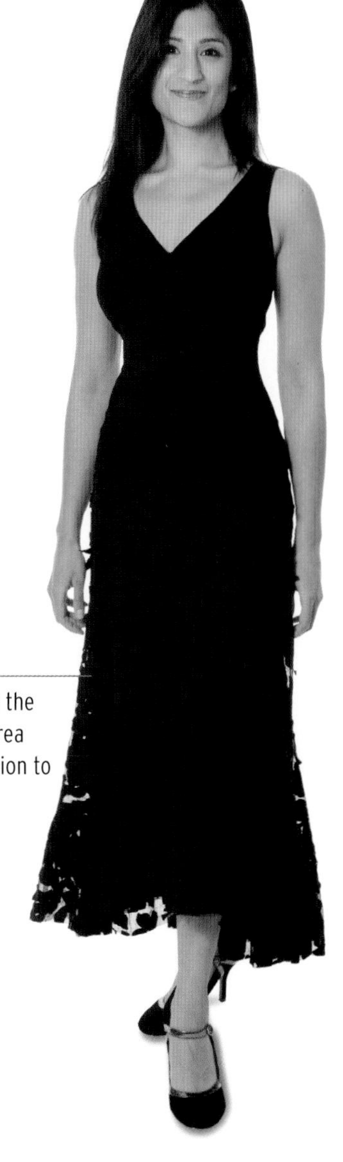

Slight flare balances the curve-hugging hip area while adding dimension to her slight frame

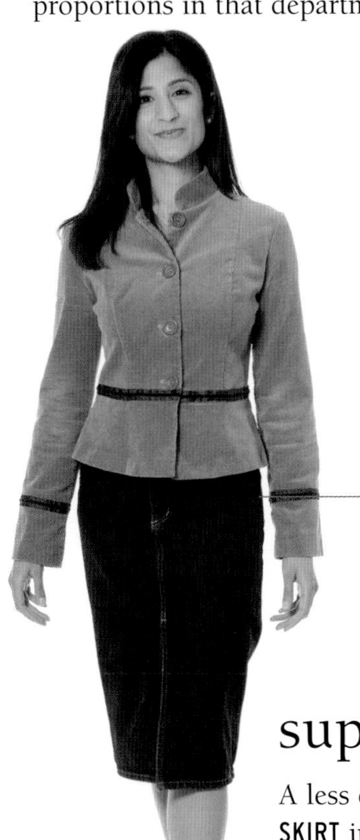

A pencil skirt shows hip and adds structure to an outfit

supriya now

A less dressy look for Supriya is this **TRADITIONAL PENCIL SKIRT** in denim. Its stiffer fabric adds the structure that Supriya's frame needs, while its shape preserves and **ENHANCES HER CURVES** to keep her overall silhouette **WELL PROPORTIONED**.

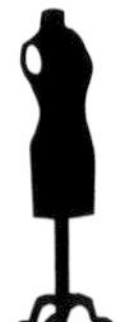

closet smarts:
SKINNY BOTTOM HALF

Deborah faces similar issues, and we see her pictured here in some bad choices, followed by two good options.

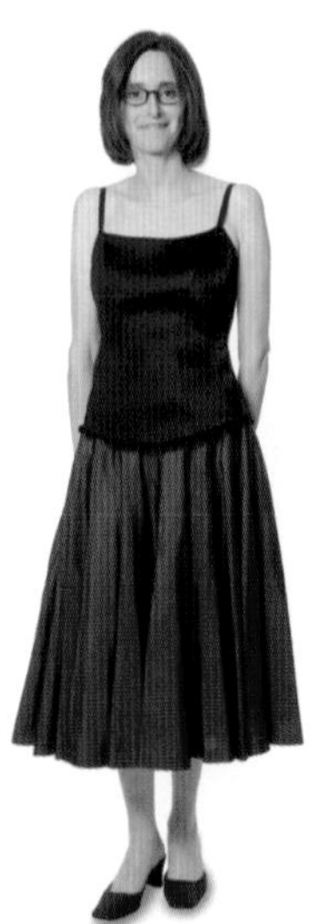

deborah before

As we saw with Supriya, Deborah's small frame runs the risk of being overwhelmed by too much fabric, and that is what we're seeing here. This skirt is too full on Deborah's frame and makes her look skinny. She can afford to add some width to her frame with fabric, but not so much that her limbs end up looking like sticks. A good alternative is a skirt with some shape to it as well as fullness, as you can see in the photo on page 165.

Silhouette is all-important.

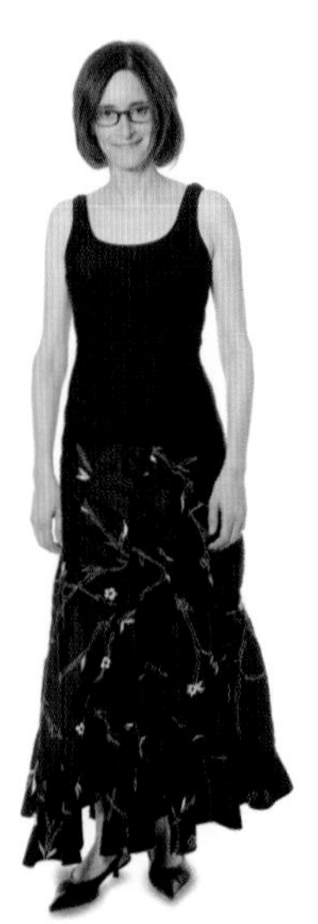

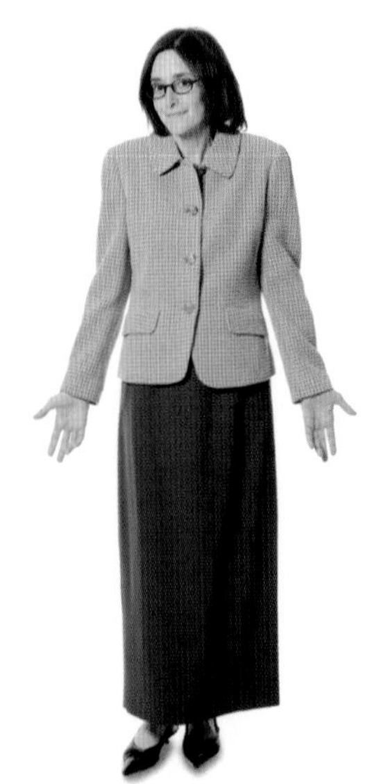

deborah before

Let me remind you that silhouette is all-important! Deborah was under the impression that a long, full skirt was the right idea to fill her out, but her selections were too full and ended up overwhelming her, as you can see in these photos. Your clothes should never give the appearance of wearing you, and that is certainly the impression we get from these skirt choices.

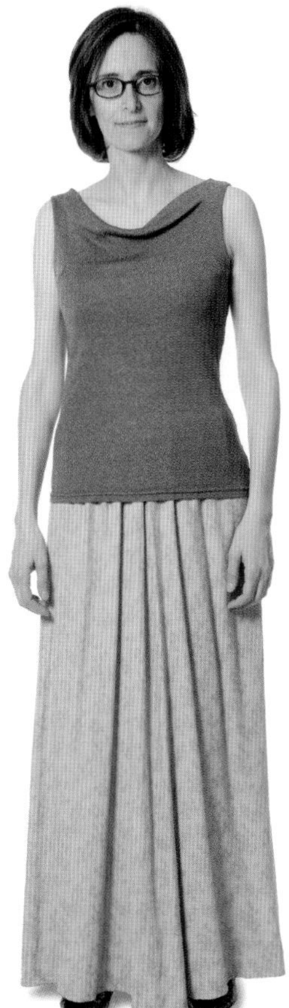

deborah now

Here, though we do fill out Deborah's frame, we still see her shape beneath (or create it) with the **CURVES** of this bias-cut skirt. Paired with a **FIGURE-HUGGING TOP** that emphasizes Deborah's curves, we get the best of both worlds. She appears more **VOLUPTUOUS** than she is, indeed **VERY SEXY AND SULTRY**, instead of like a skinny Minnie. The length helps as well. We're not left with the impression of stick legs tacked on at the bottom of her outfit.

Slight A-line adds width but does not overwhelm

deborah now

Another option for Deborah is a **SHORTER SKIRT**, which can work well for her as long as she sticks to shapes that don't emphasize the skinnier aspects of her limbs. A good short skirt option for Deborah is also one with a little shape. This skirt has a slight A-line, but one that is not so **DRAMATIC** that it creates the pendulum-leg effect that we saw pictured on Supriya's slight frame in the photo on page 162. Nonetheless, there is enough of an A here to add a little width, **SHOW A LITTLE LEG**, and, again paired with a formfitting top, **REVEAL SOME CURVES** in Deborah's figure. In this outfit she looks **SOPHISTICATED AND HIP**—well dressed rather than overdressed.

The Last Word

So, there we have it, the tricks of better skirting for all kinds of frames and figures! The various shapes and design details of skirts can work different magic on different frames, so I hope you tuned into your figure issues and can take some practical tips with you the next time you are out skimming the racks. Perhaps the simplest trick to remember, if we had to choose just one, is that A-lines work for most figures, so try on lots of them! On the other hand, bias-cut skirts pretty much work only for those with very slim hips, and that is not the majority of us, I hate to say. Those are two powerful tools to take with you to the dressing room.

For hipsters, try using the flutes and flares to proportion out the hips. And unless you are on the skinner side, watch out for fuller-cut skirts with lots of fabric, especially those that cut at the knee. And last but not least, the miniskirt just looks too girlish for most women over twenty-three. If you want to look cute, go for a funky A-line with style rather than a shorter mini. You get the same effect without looking like you are yearning to recreate your youth.

In the next and last chapter, we will take some of the basic style mantras we have learned about dressing different figures and pick a best overall look for each of our models to demonstrate—followed by an explanation of the whys and hows, of course! This will be a chance for us to review what we have learned about how to remake our silhouettes in their best image, whatever that might be.

When we are done, if you have been following me and the girls throughout, hopefully you will have the design tools to dig through your closet and evaluate your wardrobe, mixing and rematching the clothes you have now in new and more flattering combinations (and hauling some bags off to Goodwill). And I trust you'll also have the confidence you need to go out into your local dressing room with the skills to make shopping and shaping your body simpler and more pleasurable. After all, shopping shouldn't be an excruciating or confusing experience. It should be fun and creative—a chance to remake yourself and your shape every time you add a garment to your wardrobe. So, let's get to it!

ULTIMATE SKIRT STYLE

Got the skirt picture now? Take these tips with you next time you pull a skirt off the rack (or out of your closet).

1. Aim for straight As: An A-line looks good on almost every body.
2. Don't be biased: Bias-cuts draw the eye right where most of us don't want it—to all our tummy, hip, and thigh bulges.
3. The yoke's on you—or it should be! Yokes draw the eye down past the hips and drape away from the thighs.
4. Avoid frivolous fabrication: Too much fabric is . . . too much fabric on everyone, thick or thin. You don't want to *look* like you're hiding something. You want to actually hide it! Stick to skirt shapes that structure or smooth over your curves, not styles that bury them.
5. Skirting isn't everything: Girls do not live by skirts alone. Your top half should work with your skirting choices to leave an integrated overall impression. A formfitting, lower-necked top always helps to draw the eye to your décolletage and away from hip and thigh issues.

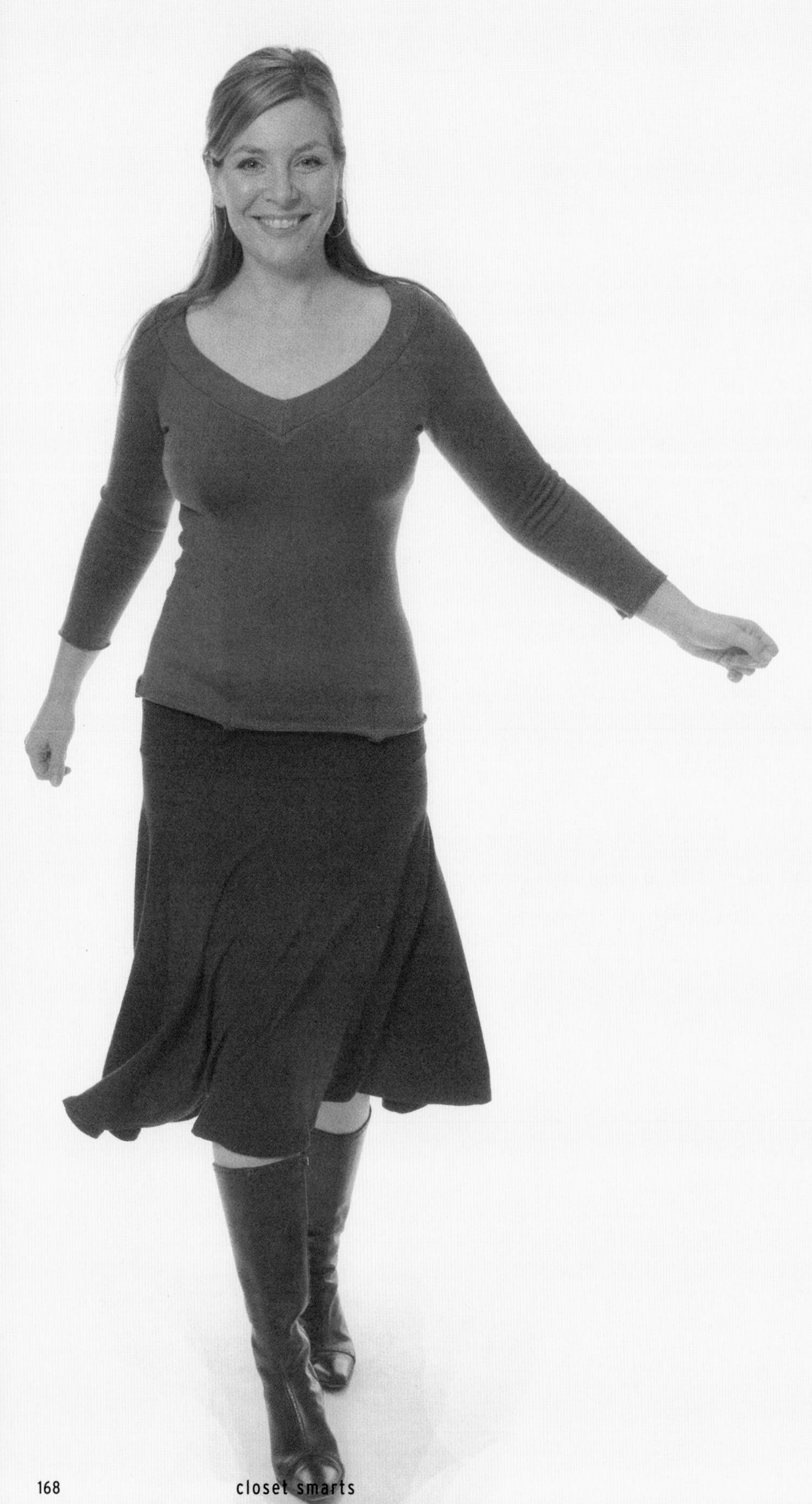

CHAPTER 10

your best look

A Flawless You

We have been on a journey across bellies and hips, over thighs and boobs, around shoulders and down to ankles, and where have we ended up? Hopefully, my mantras about sculpting your silhouette, creating two triangles, maintaining proportion throughout your outfit, and not overwhelming your frame by hiding behind clothes that are too big have stuck with you, or at least *on* you. If you've stayed with me so far, you should have a good sense at this point of which style tricks might work best to cover *your* imperfections (real or imagined), and I've given you the tools to make yourself over in your best self-image.

Finding Yourself

By now you should have a good idea how to draw attention to whatever part it is of yours that you feel most confident about. (See "Closet Smarts Style: Clothes That Fit" on the left for more on this.) If you still feel confused—or just want a refresher—here is one last chance to imbibe the most basic sense of where you can go right given your shape and size, as modeled on our gals.

In this last chapter, I want to talk to you about your overall look: how to put it together, how to present yourself through clothing, and how to look your best—all the time. We will take one more look at all of our models in a great look and talk about the hows and whys. I hope you find yourself here, and even if you end up being some combination of Felisha, Yvette, Lily, Amy, Karen, Sara, Beth, Supriya, Deborah, and Morgan, your best look is here somewhere, just waiting for you. So pick your favorite and try it on!

CLOSET SMARTS STYLE: CLOTHES THAT FIT

In my line of work, the biggest hurdle most women face in remaking themselves through dressing is letting their eyes adjust to seeing themselves in a new light. For many, this comes up most pointedly when wearing clothes that hug the body or, as I like to say, clothes that *actually fit*. I cannot stress enough to you how big an improvement this simple adjustment can make to your appearance. So, please go against your instinct to cover up. Less is truly more in this case! Show off your undeniably lovely parts, most likely your décolletage, but you know your other favorite part. Is it your butt? Your waist? Your boobs? Your ankles? Your arms? Your face? One woman's trash is another woman's treasure . . . so work it!

YVETTE: Bigger Belly, Hips, and Thighs

Yvette's got curves and a belly, but given all that we've seen throughout this book, these challenges are easy to work with to good effect. Yvette is in a position of power at work and needs to appear authoritative, but she also has a personality to boot, so no ordinary suit look is going to cut it for her. My favorite look for Yvette? This flattering combination of jacket and skirt with heels.

Why does this look work for Yvette? To begin with, like Yvette, the jacket, which is the main event of this outfit, has a lot of style and personality to it. It's great to have standout pieces in your wardrobe that actually say something about who you are and that don't make you look like everyone else. Secondly, its fabric is working for her on a number of fronts: It has some good stretch to it, so it hugs Yvette's curves, but it's also firm enough to smooth out any potential bumps through her belly area. Its cut and design also work in many ways. The racing stripes down the front both accentuate Yvette's curviness (in a flattering way) and draw the eye down the torso, elongating her midsection. Its open neck helps draw the eye to the décolletage, and its tailored cut helps sculpt Yvette's torso to the most flattering effect.

And what about Yvette's bottom half (the nether regions)? The more fluid black skirt has the effect of masking heavier hips and thighs through color and the smoothing weight of the material. The flared cut balances out Yvette's hips and shoulders to create perfect proportion head to toe. The heel adds height (always a good thing) and class.

What we see when we look at this overall look is skin in all the right places—décolletage, ankles, calves, and also Yvette's great face—and sculpting everywhere else—tummy, arms, butt, thighs, and boobs. That is what dressing your best is all about: Take control of the dubious parts, and let your best parts shine through!

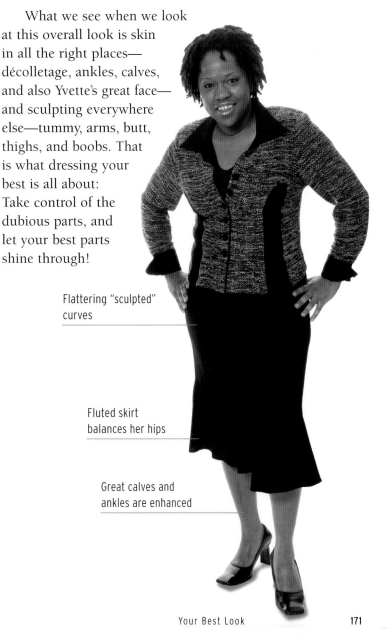

Flattering "sculpted" curves
Fluted skirt balances her hips
Great calves and ankles are enhanced

LILY: Keeping Curves in Proportion

Lily is more curvy all over, so for her, keeping her curves in proportion and creating an overall look is a main focus. She has a need for a professional polished look, but she is tired of choosing clothes that she feels wear her and leave her feeling styleless. For Lily, my favorite look has got to be this upscale casual skirt and sweater jacket ensemble.

Why? Let's start with what's showing: décolletage, calves, ankles, and face. What's sculpted? Waistline, arms, hips and thighs, butt, and bust. We use a dark-wash denim skirt here to sculpt Lily's bottom and shape it into a flattering shape. We can see the curve of her hip, but it is balanced by the slightest flare at the knee and complemented at the bottom of her silhouette with a most refined heel.

Above the waist, we are drawn to Lily's neck and face, beautifully enhanced by the pale lilac of her top, which we have layered with a refined sweater jacket. This jacket is like a miracle worker for the torso and does all the right things. It cinches just below the bust (our slimmest part), scallops over the hips, and opens up the décolletage.

What more could we ask? Lily looks shapely, lovely, and, of course, well proportioned.

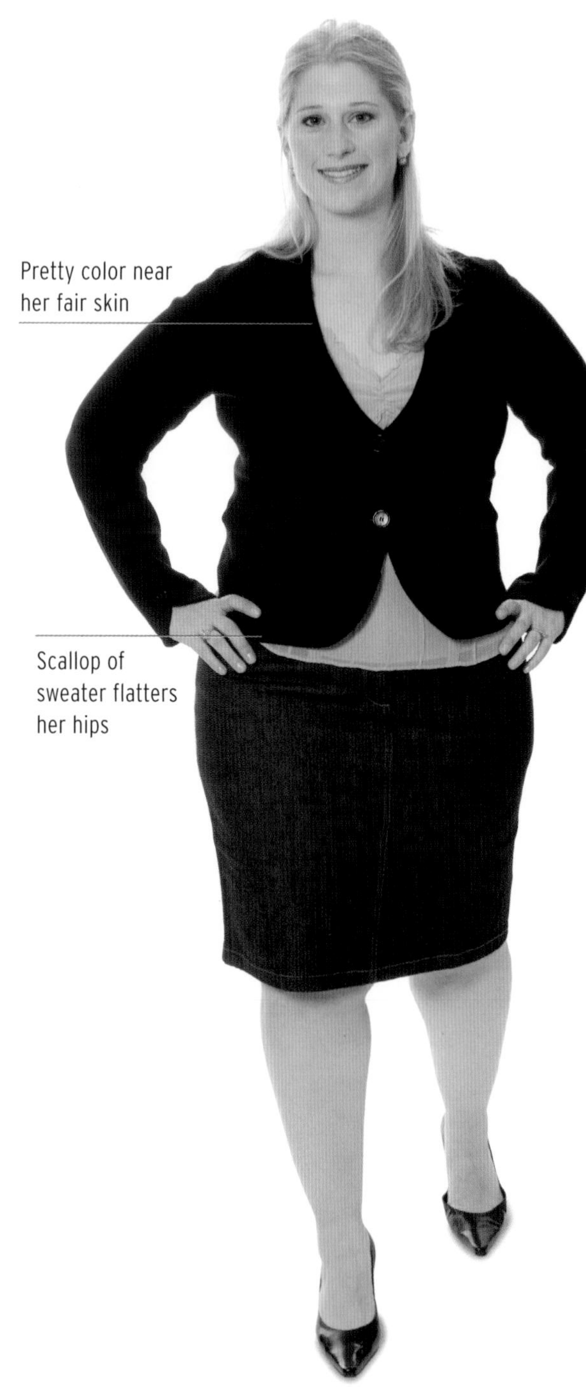
Pretty color near her fair skin
Scallop of sweater flatters her hips

Felisha: Thicker Thighs and Hips

Felisha has decided her new favorite thing to wear is skirts, and I agree, they are wondrous creatures. They can really help sculpt, de-emphasize, skirt over, and more generally take control of the shape of our bottom halves, and we could all stand to incorporate a few more of them into our wardrobes! I hope you will spend some time reviewing chapter 9 (beginning on page 149) and adding some skirts to your own closet, *soon*!

In Felisha's case, my favorite skirt look, though there were many, was this longer embroidered denim skirt paired with a body-hugging black top and black leather jacket, and, of course, refined heels.

Felisha gets all the hip and thigh coverage she wants here with the longer length of this skirt, without appearing overwhelmed in fabric due to the skirt's narrow construction. In addition, the skirt has genuine style as well as shape. Though it is longer and less curvaceous, we counteract that by pairing it with a curve-hugging and décolletage-flattering top. The sleek leather jacket gives her shoulders better proportion (in Felisha's case, it squares them off as she has more rounded shoulders). She looks as put-together as they come and sassy to boot!

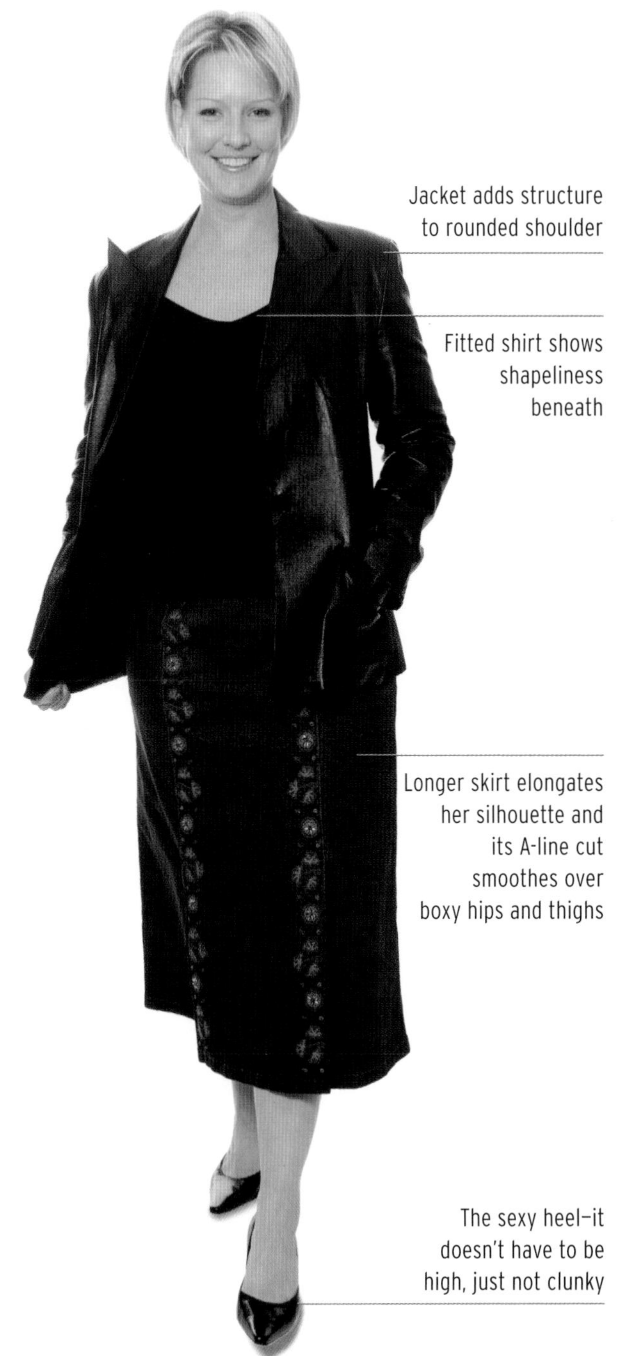
Jacket adds structure to rounded shoulder
Fitted shirt shows shapeliness beneath
Longer skirt elongates her silhouette and its A-line cut smoothes over boxy hips and thighs
The sexy heel—it doesn't have to be high, just not clunky

Amy: The Classic Hourglass

My favorite look for Amy is one we've seen before, but who can argue? There are many things you can do with an hourglass figure, because most of your proportion work has already been done. Your best bet then is to *keep* that proportion working for you. Enhancing and accentuating is the name of the game here. Certainly, do nothing that might *hide* it.

In this outfit, we use a curve-hugging top that shapes and smoothes all the torso's parts—bust, waist, tummy, and arms. We've paired it with a fluid A-line yoked skirt that smoothes over the hips and a stylish knee-high boot—all to great effect. We have simply emphasized the good and smoothed over any potential trouble spots, all while maintaining Amy's proportionally balanced silhouette. (Remember the two triangles!) Oh, that was too easy—next!

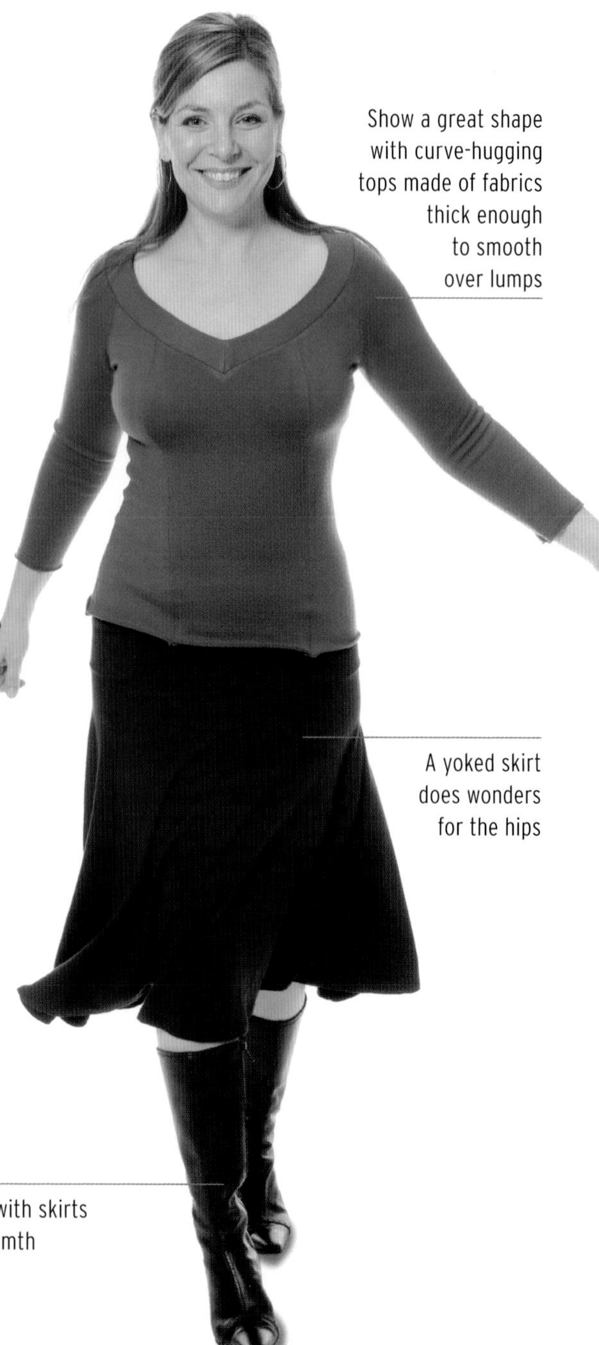

Show a great shape with curve-hugging tops made of fabrics thick enough to smooth over lumps

A yoked skirt does wonders for the hips

Full boots look great with skirts and can help with warmth in the winter

KAREN: Pearish Square

Karen! As with many of my models, there were a lot of looks we put together that I loved, so it's hard to pick just one here. We've seen Karen throughout the book in some great A-line skirts, but I think my favorite overall look for her was this layered pants option.

Karen struggles with feeling thicker through the middle and a bit square on the bottom (despite a nice flat stomach), so with this outfit, we work on both sculpting and masking. We pair nice low-waisted dark denim jeans, slightly flared at the ankle to even out her hips, with a very fitted V-neck top in a bright color. Then we cover over her torso with this stylish embroidered duster that adds both a feminine flare and some coverage for her more boyish torso.

We end up being drawn to Karen's décolletage and her beautiful face and smile, noting her nice flat tummy vis-à-vis the bright pink accent of her top, seeing nothing but lovely elongated legs (accented of course by a refined low heel), and admiring her sense of style in choice of jacket! Karen looks totally put together and oh so svelte.

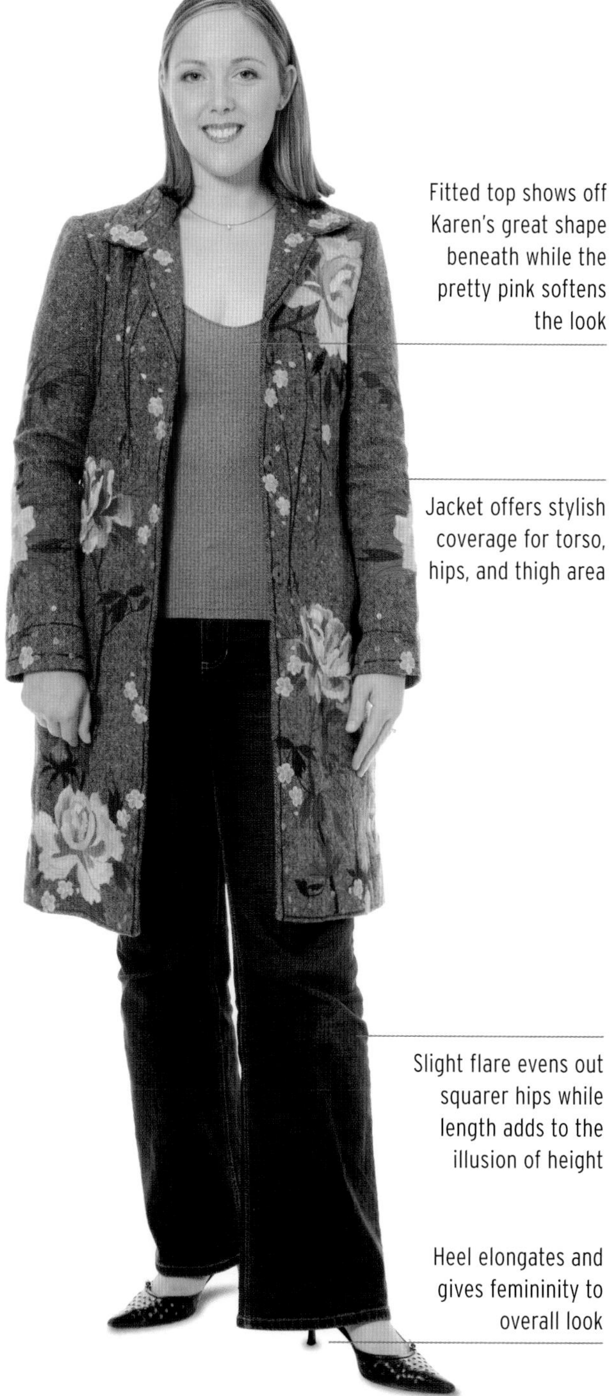

Fitted top shows off Karen's great shape beneath while the pretty pink softens the look
Jacket offers stylish coverage for torso, hips, and thigh area
Slight flare evens out squarer hips while length adds to the illusion of height
Heel elongates and gives femininity to overall look

SARA: From Boyish to Bodacious

My favorite look on Sara is this curve-accentuating skirt duet. Sara also feels that parts of her silhouette are overly square and boyish, so what better solution than to carve out some curves? They are there, but they need to be highlighted.

In this case, we rounded out Sara's shoulders with a nice Lycra and cotton top that did wonders for her bust and waist as well. By pairing it with a narrower pencil skirt that accents the curve of the hip, we got the overall effect of enhancing a very nice hourglass figure. We finished it off with a very refined pair of black slingbacks to complete the feminine look, and Sara looks as sexy as they come—no boyishness here!

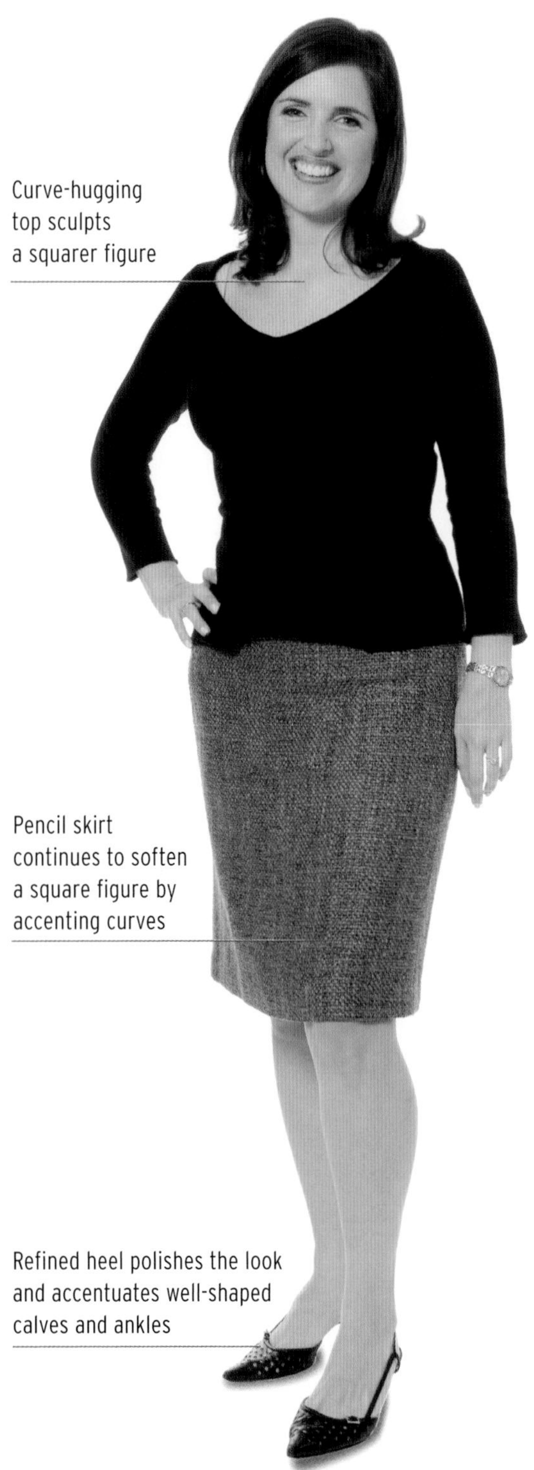

Curve-hugging top sculpts a squarer figure

Pencil skirt continues to soften a square figure by accenting curves

Refined heel polishes the look and accentuates well-shaped calves and ankles

BETH:
The Classic Pear

I picked a dress for Beth. With her butt and hips as spots of contention, empire-styled dresses really work well on her to accent her best parts and mask her sensitive ones. She could also easily pair an empire-styled top with an A-line skirt or with a low-waisted straighter-leg to bootleg-cut pants for the same effect as we have seen elsewhere in the book. But dresses, like skirts, are such an overlooked category of clothing, and one we could all stand to use to better effect in our wardrobes. They can be dressy or more casual. This one is dressy and adorable!

Beth has lovely arms and shoulders. She's very petite, but she has a wider bottom, so she needs to dress to bring her proportions into balance. This dress does the job by highlighting her best parts—shoulders, chest, décolletage, and empire waist—while flaring out over her trouble spots in a nice full, but refined, skirt.

The dress is just long enough to avoid the accusation of baby doll. Combined with a sophisticated heel, it leaves the impression that Beth, rather than being cutesy, has a real sense of sassy style. She's got great legs, and the length of the dress makes them look even longer and more delectable. Simply lovely!

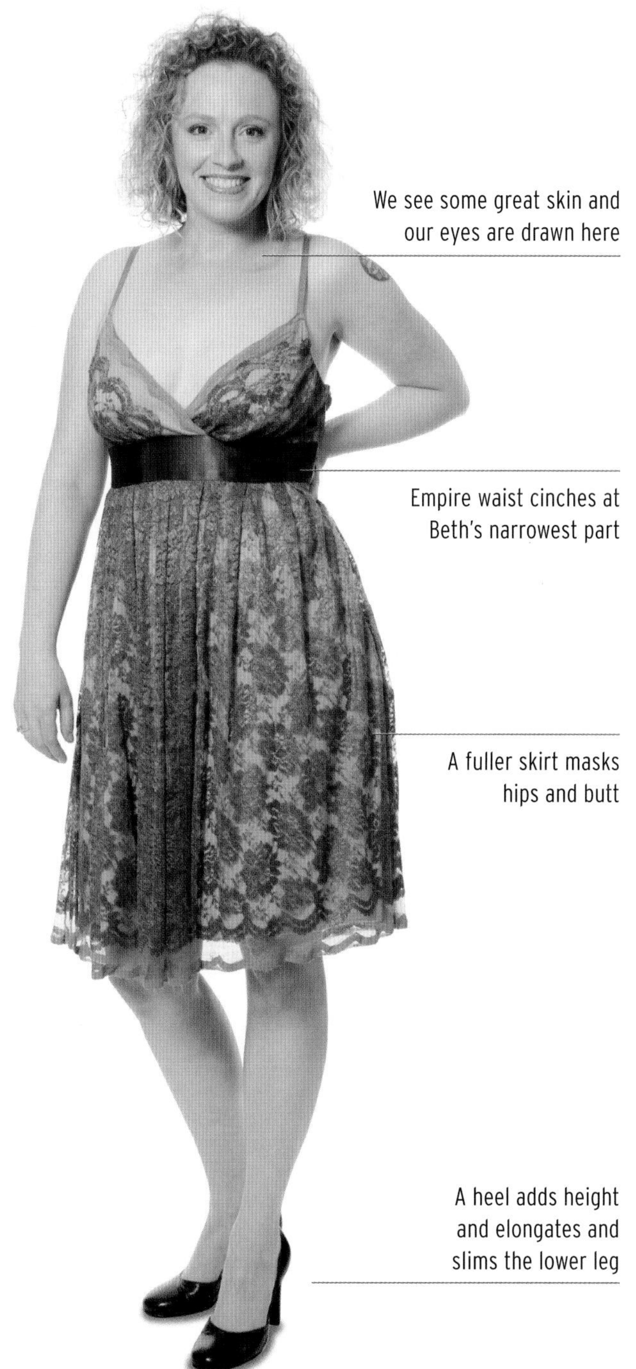

We see some great skin and our eyes are drawn here

Empire waist cinches at Beth's narrowest part

A fuller skirt masks hips and butt

A heel adds height and elongates and slims the lower leg

DEBORAH:
Skinny Minnie

One of my favorite looks for Deborah is this layering look. It takes her shape by storm and gives her figure good proportion, as well as adding a little girth to her otherwise slight frame.

Deborah can use a flared-leg pant to great effect; it adds some dimension to her little frame. She has very skinny legs, and though it's hard for her to find pants that fit, finding pants with the right *shape* is just as crucial. We used a cropped sweater here combined with a longer shirt to add some dimension and create shape throughout her torso.

The embroidered beading about the bust draws attention to her widest part (a *good* thing in her case!), drawing the eye away from her skinny arms. The overall effect is that Deborah looks taller and more lanky rather than scrawny and stick-like.

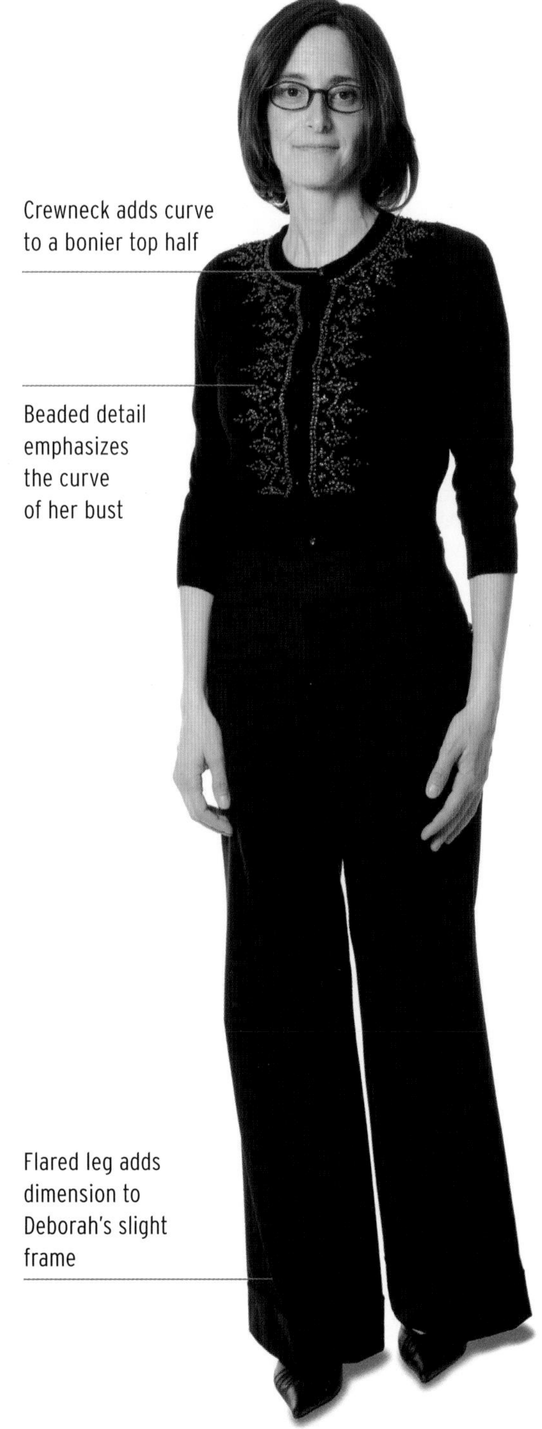

Crewneck adds curve to a bonier top half

Beaded detail emphasizes the curve of her bust

Flared leg adds dimension to Deborah's slight frame

Supriya: The Long-Waisted, Busty Skinny Minnie

I had to pick this red dress for Supriya because it looked so darn good! It also helps me emphasize some important points about reshaping her figure that are easy to copy if you have similar figure issues (long waist, big boobs, skinny limbs).

First, where are we drawn in? Supriya's décolletage, her waist, and her bust. And what have we forgotten? Her long waist, her tiny legs, and her overall skinniness? Exactly!

This dress has all the right moves. Its thicker straps fill out Supriya's shoulders and keep them from looking bony, while also highlighting her breasts without overdoing it. Its empire-styled waist draws our eyes to a nice, narrow part of her torso, while its fuller skirt conceals her long waist and adds just the right amount of fabric and flow to her figure to fill it out.

Supriya looks absolutely curvaceous in this dress, and we know from former photos that she is not. We also see just the right amount of leg, cut at just the right place (calf-length, which makes her legs look fuller rather than scrawny). Paired with a taller heel that adds height, as well as drawing the eye to a shapely calf and ankle, with this outfit we've really made Supriya over into a bodacious babe rather than anyone we might refer to as a skinny Minnie.

Though we used layering a lot throughout the book to reform Supriya's torso, a well-fashioned dress can do the same work with the right cut (empire waist and A-line). She looks absolutely perfect in this dress!

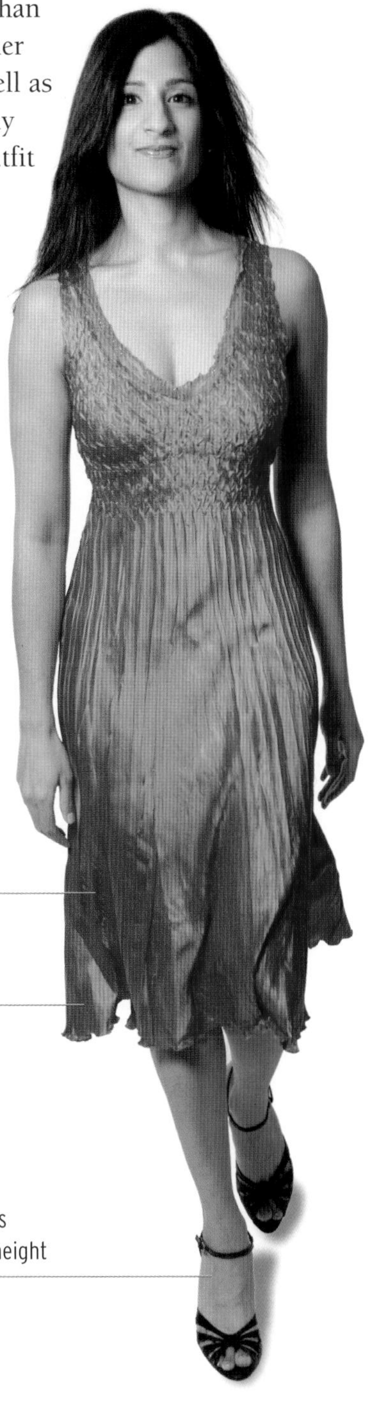

Fuller skirt adds substance to a slight frame

Hemline falls at the fullest part of her calf masking skinny legs

Heel adds needed height

Morgan: From Booty to Beauty

Last but certainly not least, I couldn't resist showing off Morgan in this fabulous dress! It does the work of thirty inferior dresses. Morgan's assets are her height, her long legs, and her overall proportions, not to mention her model good looks. But she is sensitive about her booty and thigh area, and that is where we find her best look working its hardest.

The cut of this dress does wonders for Morgan's butt and thighs. Its piping draws the eye right down to her long legs, which are emphasized even more by the asymmetrical hem of the dress. Her top is completely open, so that is where we look—at her face and chest, but not her boobs! This dress is classy and sexy with its classic black-and-white trim, and its lines are relatively safe, not overly racy. Her heels add even more height as well as the great silhouette of her calves and slim ankles. (She just needs to find a date who can compete!)

Morgan's dress works like all the best looks we have been talking about, by *emphasizing* the good, drawing attention to her best figure features, and *reshaping* the bad through design, fabric, and cut. Everyone can achieve this effect, whether you are donning a dress, a skirt, pants, or a suit.

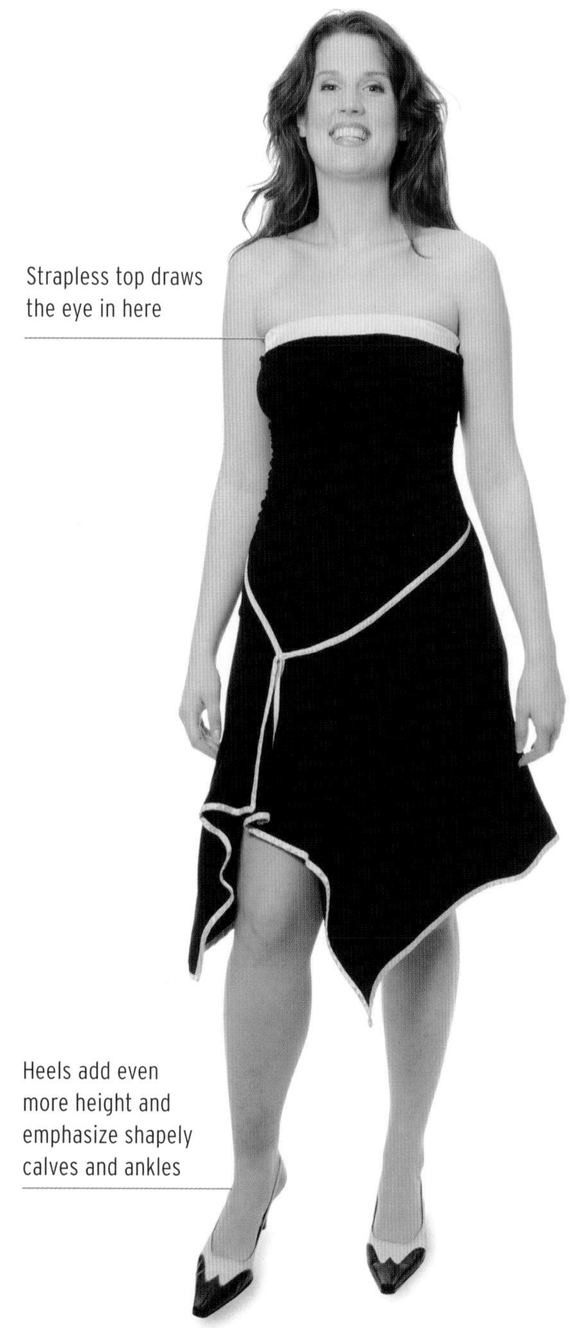

Strapless top draws the eye in here

Heels add even more height and emphasize shapely calves and ankles

The Last Word

So there they all are, women just like you, looking their best, dealing with imperfect bodies, and coming out on top. It's truly amazing what clothes can do for your shape, and there is no reason why you should not be taking full advantage of the tricks that are out there to feel better about yourself *right now*, not after you lose those elusive ten pounds. The better you feel about yourself *now*, the better the chance that you will feel motivated to do the things you want to do, while they are still worth doing!

Remember, my goal in writing this book isn't to have you throw out everything in your closet and start over. Far from it! I want to help you see your clothes—and yourself—with new eyes. Once you've analyzed your figure for its strengths and flaws, you can use the many before-and-after shots throughout the book to see how to put together the clothes you already have in new combinations, determine which garments must go, and shop with confidence to fill in your wardrobe gaps.

Take the fashion mantras from this book and get rid of the dead weight in your closet now! It's time to start dressing your best every day.

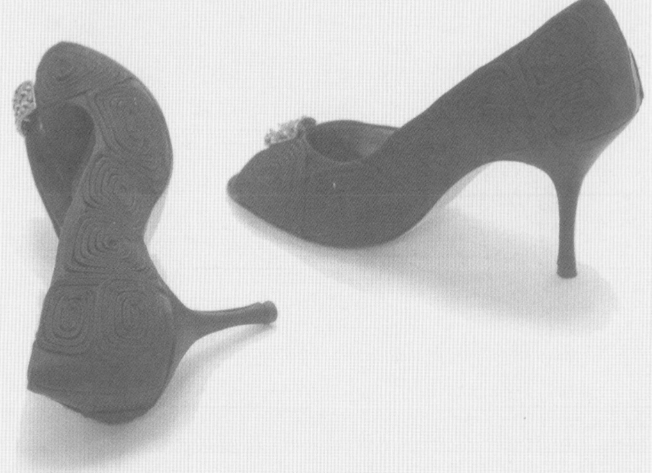

EMILY'S ULTIMATE FASHION MANTRAS

If I had to sum up this entire book's worth of wisdom on a single page, the ten points below —my fashion mantras—are what I'd want to tell you. I suggest that you photocopy this list and tape it to the inside of your closet door, so you'll be reminded to use your Closet Smarts every time you get dressed. And don't forget to make a second copy to take along when you head out to the stores!

1. Start with a good knowledge of your shape and a good idea of what shape you want to achieve. (Remember that image of two triangles that meet at the tips where your waist would be and aim for that.)
2. The number one goal you should try to achieve through dressing is creating good proportion from your shoulders through your waist and hips down to your ankles. No matter what your clothing size, if you create a well-proportioned silhouette, you will always look your best.
3. Always look for clothes that actually have shape. This means design details like darts at the bust and torso, yokes, refined hems, flared and boot legs, etc.
4. Material can make a big difference when you are creating a silhouette. The stiffer the fabric, the more sculpting a piece can do for your figure. A little stretch (Lycra) is also a boon in this department. It helps accentuate curves and shapeliness while smoothing out the lumps and bumps.
5. Use design tricks to effectively mask your trouble zones or even out your proportions–things like ruching, V-necks, empire waists, wrap tops, scalloped hems, fluted or ruffled hems, flat fronted trousers, busy prints, etc.
6. Less is always more! Opt for clothes that show more and hug your body more closely. (You can control that hug with tips 3 through 5 above.) When you wear clothes that are too big, you just look like you are hiding something, and it's never flattering to swathe yourself in too much fabric.

7. Simpler is better, as a general rule. Stay focused on the shape of your silhouette and work with basic, more neutral classics as you start out. Don't get overly complicated in your look. You'll make fewer mistakes if your look is simpler, and you'll get better at dressing your unique shape.
8. Don't decide ahead of time that you can never wear a certain color. Experiment liberally, and you will surely surprise yourself once in a while.
9. Same goes for what you actually will and won't wear. Since Katharine Hepburn made it okay for women to wear pants and suits, most women totally underutilize skirts and dresses. You may think they are not for you, but I dare you to see yourself with new eyes and try some on! They can be great for casual and professional wear, as well as for dressier occasions.
10. Last but not least, make every fashion choice count and make every day a "best outfit" day. If there is anything in your wardrobe that makes you feel mediocre, get rid of it. If it doesn't contribute to the principles we have outlined in this book, it's not working for you. Clothes are your tools, not your enemy. All that's left to do is use them to best effect!

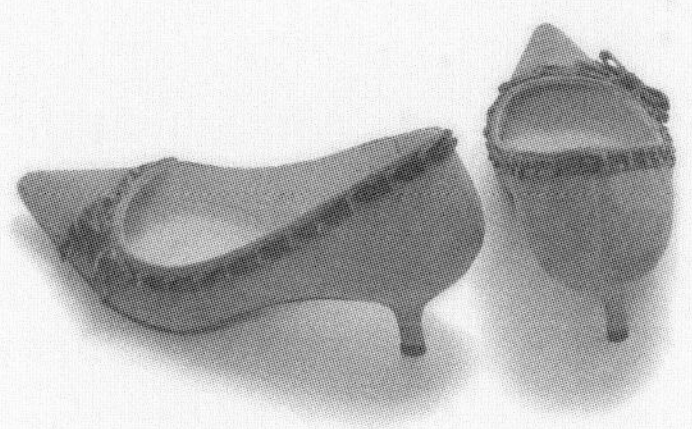

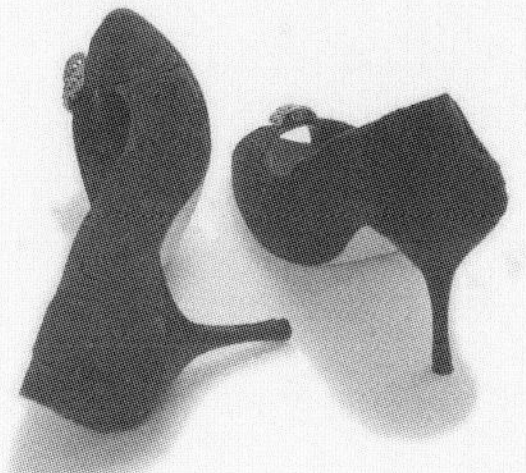

your turn

I wish I could meet each and every one of you and rework your closets with you. But I have done my best to get you started with this pictorial of how to achieve your best looks and create your best shape. Now it's your turn. How do you really get started, then?

BUY A FULL-LENGTH MIRROR

First and foremost, please make sure you have a full-length mirror near your closet. I cannot tell you how many people avoid having to face whether their outfits actually make sense or are fashion disasters by not having one. This is also the best way to avoid investing in your shoe wardrobe. I guess the idea is that what you can't see won't hurt you! Sorry, but that's not gonna fly with me (your new personal stylist in print). No more of those clunky, salt-marked, worn out, dated shoes that are practical for all that walking you do and those snowy and rainy days. But I digress (we'll get to that in the next book). Get yourself a full-length mirror!

SORT YOUR CLOTHES BY TYPE AND COLOR

Next? Sort your clothes by type and color. Start with the bottom pieces (skirts and pants—I pray you don't have any shorts, or at least that they are not hanging in your closets). Next, sort your dresses, then your tops, again, also by color (short sleeve, long sleeve, jackets). Separate any suits you have hanging together. There's a whole skirt and jacket there, surely you can wear them separately on different occasions, yes? Take all those bulky ski sweaters your mother knit you out of your closet now! Save that top shelf (or a hanging shelf bag) for your more refined sweaters, also sorted by color. Aahhh. Now you can see what you have.

TRY ON WHAT YOU HAVE

Next? Play dress-up! Try what you have on and be brutally honest with yourself. If there is any excuse that comes to mind as to why you have hung onto something despite the fact that you never wear it (its has a funny flap, it clings weirdly on my hips, the length is kinda off), get rid of it! As long as you have that thought about it, you will always put it on and take it off again. So why is it taking up space? Everything hanging in your closet should make you feel good when you put it on, or at least act as a neutral building block for a good outfit.

MAKE NEW COMBINATIONS

You may need a friend (or me) to help you with the next step. Try putting things together in a new way, such as pairing that suit jacket you only ever wear with its matching pants or skirt with some dark denim jeans and a little heel. Put that silk shell under a stylish cardigan and a more casual skirt with a pair of tall boots. Mix pink and brown, teal and gray, dark red and mauve. One thing I have discovered in every woman's closet I have gotten into is that there is a lot more there than you think there is, and before you go out shopping, you need to get really familiar with what you have, how to use it to best effect, and then and only then, how to build on it.

MAKE TIME AND DO IT!

If I can give you one bit of advice at the start of your new style adventures—and you bought this book, so I know you care—why not carve out a few hours to do this for yourself? Stay in some Saturday night instead of going out, take a day off from work, hire a babysitter, and send your spouse or partner out with friends. Then open a bottle of wine, or brew a pot of coffee, or grab a giant sized bottle of water, and act like your closet is your own private boutique.

This can be fun, and even if it's work, it's the kind of work with the biggest pay-off. It's like mowing a lawn and looking back over at the beautiful peacefulness you have created. It will give you peace of mind, and at the very least, it will garner you some great outfit ideas for the next week. Ultimately, going through this process will give you a very solid (and much-needed) idea of who you are, where you came from, and where you want to go. And those are the facts, ma'am.

UNLEASH YOUR INNER GLAMOURPUSS

I know there is a glamourpuss waiting to emerge in there. She is sultry and stylish, polished and put together, sassy and smart, classy and chic, or trendy and tart. Are you one of these? Don't you want to be? Stop mourning the loss of your twenty-something figure and start making the most of the one you have. You have absolutely nothing to lose. Believe it. Do it. Be her, the one everyone always says looks so put-together and intentional about her look. She's waiting for you in your closet!

index

index

index

ACKNOWLEDGMENTS

I never thought I'd hear myself saying this (or writing it as the case may be), but it's true: Writing a book is not a solitary achievement. It is the result of a pretty major network of people: friends, colleagues, editors, family, and sometimes even random people you meet on the street. In this case, first and foremost, I could not have written this book without being lucky enough to rope my photographer friend, Liz Linder, into working on it with me. Not only is she the consummate image maker in so many different genres of photography, but she is a wonderful friend and a tireless worker, and I could not have done this without her. Same goes for her studio manager, Casey Engels, who was more patient with me than I ever deserved and who dealt with some hairy math equations as we numbered and renumbered the photos for the book!

Secondly, though hardly secondly, I have my models to thank—all of whom volunteered their time and their bodies, for my project—even after finding out that there would be underwear photos of them distributed nationally for all to see. The models were brave, flexible, funny, and professional, and they have all become my friends if they were not before. I admire each and every one of them, and I thank them from the bottom of my heart. Here's to you Amy Bebergal, Beth Daly, Felisha Foster, Lily Leaton, Supriya Mehta, Karen Santospago, Morgan Stockmayer, Deborah Wieder, Yvette Wilkes, and Sara Wilkinson.

To the ladies at LOOKS Boutique (my second family) in Cambridge: Ellen, MaryBeth, Paige, and Suzanne, for their help with the clothes. And especially to LOOKS' owner, Judy Armell, who gave me free access to her store's wonderful clothes for my shoots and also pretty much acts as my "other" mother in so many ways.

To my editor Ellen Phillips, for being so patient with me and for her keen eye at pulling out the important points in my long-winded prose to highlight for all of you readers.

To the women in my entrepreneurial group WREN (Women's Roundtable Entrepreneurial Network): Karen A., Abbey K., Hannah, Nancy, Sheila, Ellen, Liz, and Sonja, for continuing to inspire me and keep me going in many senses.

And to my family (Mom, Dad, Hurtt, Sarah, Carrie, Amy, Peter, and Jimmy, Pat C., and David J.) for supporting me and believing in me always, despite my changing life paths. And for my boys, Noah and Theo, the lights of my life.

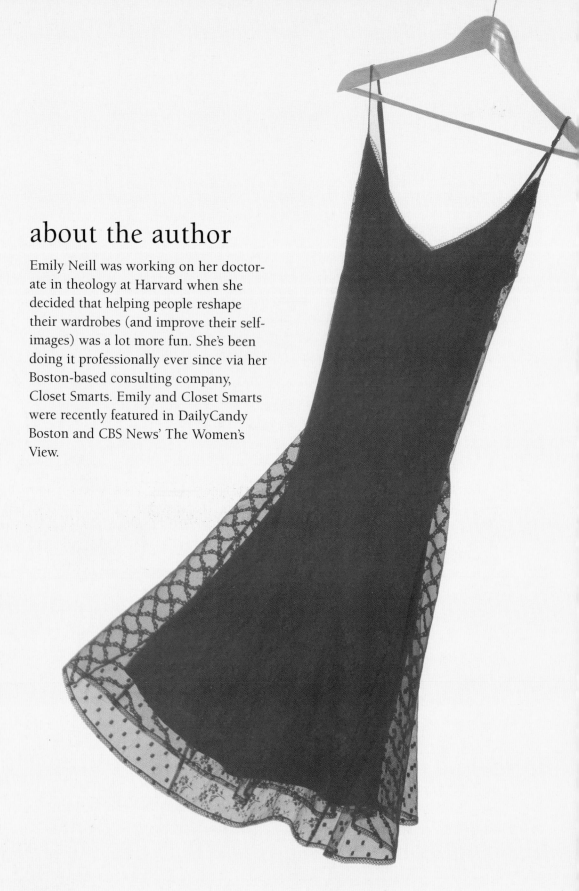

about the author

Emily Neill was working on her doctorate in theology at Harvard when she decided that helping people reshape their wardrobes (and improve their self-images) was a lot more fun. She's been doing it professionally ever since via her Boston-based consulting company, Closet Smarts. Emily and Closet Smarts were recently featured in DailyCandy Boston and CBS News' The Women's View.